The 8 Colors of Fitness

Discover Your Color-Coded Fitness Personality
and Create an Exercise Program You'll Never Quit!

Suzanne Brue

Suzanne Brue

Foreword by Katharine D. Myers

Oakledge Press, Delray Beach
April 2008

© 2008 by Suzanne Brue
Published by Oakledge Press, Delray Beach, Florida

The names of some interview subjects have been changed to preserve their privacy.

ISBN-13: 978-0-9795625-0-1

Library of Congress Control Number: 2007908282

First Edition, First Printing

For Nord

TABLE OF CONTENTS

THANKS

Many people were instrumental in the writing of this book, and I would like to extend my gratitude to all of them. First, I wish to thank all the people I interviewed. They cheerfully submitted to my interrogations about their exercise preferences, sharing their fitness stories in person, on the phone, via e-mail, or by responding to a questionnaire on my website. They were always available for follow-up as my research prompted the need for additional information.

Once I had my data, I was lucky to find just the right people at every stage of writing this book. While I believed that the stories I gathered "told themselves," the job of putting them on paper was ahead of me. I could not have done so without the unflagging efforts of Pat Goudey O'Brien. Together we wrestled with the many ways to organize these stories into a narrative. Pat, a talented writer and committed writing partner, always responded to changes as an opportunity for additional clarity and greater precision. She kept the big picture in mind, invaluable for me as I could find myself easily lost in the data. Pat always went the extra mile —including several late nights and even an occasional all-nighter.

At the next stage, Lauren Starkey was the right person to refine the work and take it from manuscript to book. As an avid exerciser (and former fitness instructor) as well as a writer and editor, Lauren "got it" immediately. She knew what had to be done and with skill and Intuition carried it to the next level. I could now see the book taking form. Our partnership was so gratifying.

Sue Ducharme magically appeared to carry the book across the finish line. Her skillful proofreading and helpful editorial comments were just what were needed to prepare it for publication.

I am also deeply indebted to many professional colleagues in the Myers-Briggs/ Jungian community who so graciously and generously shared their time and insights as I explored this new application of psychological type. Their interest, encouragement, and feedback were invaluable.

Special thanks to two individuals from the medical and fitness fields. Dr. Liana Lianov, Director of the Healthy Lifestyles Division of The American Medical Association, carefully read an early manuscript and suggested potential applications in the health field. Jim Mizes, CEO of Club One, suggested a number of revisions that made this book more user friendly for coaches, trainers, and others working in the fitness industry.

My gratitude to some special friends, whose interest in this project was unfailing. They enthusiastically supported me during the six years I spent on my research and writing: Iris Benjamin, Jill Gutknecht, Don Kjelleren, Dee Pomerleau, Rissa Seigneur, and Kevin Veller.

And finally, thank-you to my incredible family who cheered me on every step of the way: Alexia Brue, Erik Brue, Marget Brue, Ethan Klemperer, Hanna Brue, Nora Brue, Carolyn Off, Catheryn Brue, Leslie Brue, Ruby Brue, Trent Watts, Russell Watts, and my mom, Doris Watts. Special thanks to my brother, Ronny Watts, not only for his support with the book, but also for graciously allowed me to tag along and enjoy his years with the Boston Celtics. (And Ronny, thanks for doing your best to make sure I wouldn't "throw like a girl.") To my husband, Nord—your enthusiasm, interest, and contributions to this entire project made it so much more fun!

Why do so many people start exercise programs and fail to maintain them? In *The 8 Colors of Fitness*, Suzanne Brue applies principles of Jungian psychological type to address this question.

Suzanne is an expert practitioner in the use of the Myers-Briggs Type Indicator® assessment (MBTI) and has in-depth knowledge of the Jungian personality theory on which the Indicator is based. A chance conversation triggered her to wonder if a personality type influences people's preferences for the kind of exercise they find satisfying.

Her findings, resulting from six years of focused exploration, form the basis of *The 8 Colors of Fitness: Discover Your Color-Coded Fitness Personality and Create an Exercise Program You'll Never Quit!* The patterns she discovered demonstrate that the answer to her question is a resounding *Yes!*

The information provided will prove to be of valuable assistance to individuals, as well as personal trainers, physical therapists, and medical specialists, in designing programs that each person is most likely to maintain. Eight chapters describe the characteristics of each group, and a separate chapter addresses tips for professionals.

The 8 Colors of Fitness is well-written and user-friendly in organization. During workshops with the author prior to publishing, I found her excitement at what she was finding and its potential for leading individuals to exercise they would enjoy and maintain both energizing and engaging. She conveys that positive energy in her writing—it is contagious.

Her approach—grouping the sixteen types into eight pairs—is thoughtful and appropriate to her findings. At first I was puzzled at the selection of a color for each grouping. Now I find it adds a useful and creative dimension in revealing the core quality of each group. Examples: ISTJ's and ISFJ's are True Blues (Tried and True); ESTP's and ESFP's are Roaring Reds (Now!); INTP's and INFP's are Saffrons Seeking (Making Workouts into Play). I delight both in being a Saffron and in the affirmation that the criteria "Fun" is reason enough for my choices.

The history of the MBTI has been one

of ongoing additions to its areas of application: careers, personal counseling, learning and teaching, team development, etc. Brue has pioneered a new dimension: exercise and the individual differences of type. I have found that this new perspective has enriched and deepened my understanding of each type in a fresh and rewarding way—this after 65 years of familiarity with Jungian personality type and the MBTI. Valuable learning!

Katharine D. Myers
The Myers-Briggs®Trust
2007

INTRODUCTION

This book began with a casual conversation with my mother in the spring of 2001. (Thanks, Mom.) At the time, she was coping with a torn rotator cuff, and she described her visits to a physical therapist. My mother is an outgoing and friendly woman, and, true to type, she'd developed a personal relationship with the therapist, who gave her individual attention and positive feedback.

As she discussed her exercises with me, I recognized how specific her descriptions were—comments such as "I like to know exactly what I'm doing," "I like things spelled out," and "I want to make sure that I'm doing it correctly" peppered her speech. These expressions were familiar to me from a lifetime of conversations with her.

Concrete details have always assured my mother and guided her decisions. Even today, whether talking about locking the door to her apartment when I leave or about using her washing machine, my mom always states and restates the steps I should follow. These instructions are often backed up with examples of some catastrophe that befell a neighbor or friend who was not careful. Is it is any wonder that for her, in the context of physical therapy and exercise, specific and safe procedures, as well as personal connections, are paramount?

As I began to connect my mother's personality with her approach to exercise, I was curious about how she viewed other experiences with activity and sports over her lifetime. For many years, she played doubles tennis regularly. She spoke of loving the game, particularly the camaraderie with friends. Playing tennis was primarily a social activity, she said, not exercise. In addition, she and my dad played golf with friends, an activity she also described as social.

Shortly after these initial observations, I spoke with a close friend whose personality reminded me of my mother's. Iris is a jazz singer and a music booking agent who equates physical exercise with suffering, something she must endure to mitigate her osteoporosis. Over lunch, Iris said that she'd recently joined a gym, which she noted was cleaner, smaller, and friendlier than her former gym. In describing the staff, Iris said, "They know me, really care, and treat me as an individual." Her sense of personal connection reminded me of my mother's response to trainers and teachers. Iris had high hopes that the new gym environment and friendly staff would increase her motivation to lift weights and continue to engage in aerobics.

I realized that my mother and Iris shared a set of Myers-Briggs Type Indicator (MBTI®) preferences. (I'll discuss MBTI in Chapter One.) In the parlance of type, they're both ESFJs. Their stories brought to mind another friend of the same type. Dee, an artist and professional game designer, rarely exercised at all until she reached her mid-forties, when she arranged to work with a personal trainer three mornings a week. The trainer (who quickly became a friend) designed Dee's program and remained at her side the entire time, monitoring her weights, adjusting resistance levels on the treadmill and bike, and providing positive feedback. On a nice day, they would go for a walk together, chatting amiably.

I was intrigued by the patterns I saw in these women who shared ESFJ preferences for personal relationships with their trainers, step-by-step instructions, and assurances regarding safety and correct form. When I realized how alike they were, I decided to explore whether other types shared preferences in their approaches to exercise and physical fitness.

Informally, I began questioning colleagues and friends who exercised regularly, and significant patterns emerged. In light of these patterns, I realized that comments in popular culture relating to exercise and personality didn't necessarily ring true. The common advice seemed more like conjecture than solid information. Suggestions such as, "If you're an Extravert, find an exercise buddy" didn't hold up. What's the function of an exercise buddy? Do all Extraverts want one? What about Introverts—could they benefit from having a buddy?

I searched for more information on the connection between personality type and physical exercise in the body of MBTI literature, as well as in popular books, but found little. That was more than six years ago. Since then, I have asked the question: How does the personality variable influence exercise patterns, approaches, and motivation? Why do some people engage in physical activity year after year while others, in spite of their best intentions, do not? During hundreds of interviews, I began learning how fit and physically active people of each of the sixteen MBTI types maintained their exercise programs.

My investigations were based on the belief that a key to identifying sustainable exercise rests with understanding our natural energy and our preferences in terms of approach and motivation. Motivation to exercise can be complex and may include components such as culture, family, friends, finances, and health. It is not the intention of this book to reduce the complexity of exercise choices to one variable—rather, the element of personality is the focus of my work and the subject of this book.

The research for this book is based on hundreds of interviews, as well as self-reported data, addressing common aspects of physical exercise including motivation, approach, focus, preferred environments, interpersonal connections, and preferred coaching styles. I used a questionnaire designed in consultation with a professor of research methodology at the University of Vermont (see Fig. 2.1, p. 17). Subjects from each of the sixteen MBTI types came from all walks of life and various age groups. While my research was done primarily in the United States, respondents from Canada, England, Sweden, Egypt, and New Zealand participated.

I also learned from and relied upon self-completed questionnaires returned by visitors to my Web site (www.suzannebrue. com) as well as feedback from individ-

uals who participated in my workshops or attended my presentations. In addition, I interviewed personal trainers, physical therapists, coaches, and a variety of medical professionals concerning their observations on patterns of exercise.

From my own experience, I recognize that physical activity has always been an easy element to include in my life—I typically exercise an hour a day, five or six days a week. I struggle with many things in life; I have never struggled with exercise. I started swimming laps in a pool in 1980 and have been physically active on a consistent basis ever since. It became a necessity, even with three young children and a busy work schedule.

I don't believe I'm necessarily more motivated than non-exercisers. I believe I was fortunate to stumble on activities that worked *with* my personality, and I've enjoyed the benefits. Through my research I began to understand *why* that was. Now I want to share that understanding with you.

In retrospect, it's not surprising that I picked up on my mother's comments about her exercises. I had become fascinated with the Myers-Briggs Type Indicator, which I used for over a decade in my work as a career counselor and Director of the Pre-

Medical Advising Program at the University of Vermont. My mother's comments sparked a new opportunity to combine a professional pursuit with a personal passion for fitness.

My intention in writing this book is to help people to understand their most effective approaches to physical exercise. I have chosen to ground this new application in a color framework that resonates with each type—thus The 8 Colors of Fitness program. It is designed to identify individual "exercise personalities," and by doing so help people find ways to realistically and conveniently integrate exercise into their lives.

This continues to be a fascinating opportunity for me to work with the Jung/Myers model of personality type and to apply it to the study of physical activity and exercise choices. It is my hope that you, too, will find this information interesting and helpful as you search for ways to make regular physical activity a more natural part of your life.

Suzanne Brue
December, 2007

SECTION ONE

The Foundation

CHAPTER 1

A Short Primer on Personality Type

Burlington, Vermont, January 1998

The table was long and handsomely set. The stately dining room at Englesby House, residence of the president of the University of Vermont, was filled with the evening's guests. In academic communities, invitations to dine at the president's house are highly prized, even though people expect more formality than fun.

Polite conversation during the meal ranged from weighty topics of world affairs to recent academic offerings before it settled on an entertaining discussion of proverbs, those epigrams of folk wisdom that help us to understand and guide our lives.

The "professor of proverbs"—Wolfgang Meider, UVM's world-acclaimed expert and the author of more than one hundred books and monographs on this form of folklore—talked about proverbs that preserved a nation (Lincoln's), that saved the Western world (Churchill's), and that reflected a nation's mood (Truman's).

I sat quietly, listening. When there was a lull in the conversation, I spoke up. "Wolfgang," I said. "What's your favorite proverb?"

It seemed a safe question, as the peace had been won, the world had already been saved, and the national mood was optimistic. Why shouldn't we hear what this learned man considered the most engaging bit of wisdom from all that he'd come upon during his years in the field?

Professor Meider didn't miss a beat. "That's easy," he said. "*Different strokes for different folks.* If you know that, you get everything."

Different strokes for different folks: five simple words that form a fundamental statement about human nature. When Professor Meider spoke them at the president's table, I was taken by surprise—not because I'd never heard the saying before—of course I had. What amazed me was that he had distilled into five familiar words the essence of a subject that has been at the center of my professional life for fifteen years—namely, the study of human nature and our differing personalities and preferences. And he included a critical addendum: "If you know that, you get everything."

Those five words form the basis of type theory and, consequently, of this book. They imply a two-step process: first, recognize that we all have preferences, and second, understand the nature and expression of those individual preferences, or "strokes."

What does this have to do with the study of physical activity and exercise? Everything.

FROM KABBALA TO SHAKESPEARE TO PERSONALITY TYPE THEORY

Self-knowledge is the first step—some might argue the most important step—in making good decisions. This notion isn't a recent invention of New Age self-help gurus. Its underlying truth was appreciated as far back as the Greek civilization that built the temple for the Oracle at Delphi with the words *Know Thyself* inscribed over the entrance. The ancient Kabbalists introduced the maxim into Hebrew in the thirteenth century as a tenet of their mystical practice. It is echoed again in *Hamlet*, when Shakespeare's character Polonius counsels his son, "To thine own self be true."

A modern-day framework for "knowing thyself" is the Myers-Briggs Type Indicator®, an instrument used to measure individual differences and describe varieties of personality. It is adapted from the work of Swiss psychiatrist C. G. Jung, who wrote *Psychological Types* in the early twentieth century.

Katharine Briggs and her daughter Isabel Myers studied Jung's work and were intrigued by the potential they saw for the widespread, practical application of his theories. Building on their early research with nursing and medical students, Briggs and Myers developed the MBTI to identify personality preferences (or "types"), intending to make Jung's concepts accessible to the broader public. Seventy years later, the MBTI has developed into the most widely used personality descriptor in the world. It has been translated into twenty-one languages, is employed in cultures around the globe, and is taken in various forms by more than five million people each year.

With more than half a century of research behind it, the MBTI enjoys wide acceptance in the public sector and in industry, where it is applied in organizational development, leadership, conflict management, team dynamics, career counseling, education, and communication arenas.

But while the MBTI distinguishes sixteen distinct personality types, it is nonjudgmental. That is to say, no type or types are better than or preferred over the others. All types are equally valuable. By identifying your type, you gain an understanding that has practical applications and you can use that knowledge to improve many areas of your life, from relationships to careers, health programs to fitness regimens.

DETERMINING PERSONALITY TYPES

Myers and Briggs determined that identifying one's type begins with an understanding of the four dimensions, or dichotomies, of personality.

According to the model, individuals energized primarily by the world of other people, places, and things are *Extraverts*, indicated by *E*. Those who turn more often to their inner world for energy (even though they may be highly social) are *Introverts,* indicated by *I* (see Fig. 1.1, page 6).

The second dichotomy looks at how people gather information about themselves and perceive the world. Some individuals tend to seek out hard facts and sensory data that they experience directly. Naturally aware of the physical sensations in and around them, their Perceiving preference is *Sensing,* indicated by *S*. Others trust flashes of insight, musing over ideas and abstractions, and focusing on the big picture. They lean toward *Intuition,* indicated by *N* (to avoid confusion with I for Introversion).

In the same manner, the third dichotomy sorts Judging or decision-making preferences in terms of *Thinking* or *Feeling*. Both types are rational, but the decision process in individuals with a preference for *Thinking* (indicated by *T*) tends to be more detached and analytical; those with a preference for *Feeling*

Because we all seek out situations that allow us to use our best skills, knowing our type can help us to understand why we negotiate reality the way we do.

—Lenore Thompson, *Personality Type, An Owner's Manual* (1998) (indicated by *F*) tend to be more personal and empathic.

Finally, some people prefer to engage with the world in an information-gathering mode; others prefer to emphasize decision-making. Those who extend the information-gathering period, keeping their options open longer, exhibit a preference for *Perceiving,* indicated by *P.* Those who prefer to engage the world with decisiveness and a desire for closure exhibit a preference for *Judging,* indicated by *J.*

These eight preferences can be arranged into sixteen distinct groupings, forming the sixteen MBTI type codes that identify normal personalities based on preferences for Extraversion/Introversion, Sensing/ Intuition, Thinking/Feeling, and Judging/ Perceiving. A chart describing the sixteen types is shown in Figure 1.2 (see pages 12-13).

USING ALL, PREFERRING SOME

At times an individual who has a preference for Intuition may rely on sensory data for information, just as someone with a Judging preference might decide mid-course to change direction as new facts emerge. In other words, we employ all eight dimensions or dichotomies of personality from time to time. However, each person has four that are preferred.

A frequently used method aimed at letting people experience the difference between their preferred and non-preferred functions is the following handwriting exercise. On the line below, write your name with your preferred hand.

_____

Most people say that writing with their preferred hand feels natural, easy, and comfort-

FIGURE 1.1 The Four Dichotomies

Where is your natural source of energy?
(E) Extraversion------------------I------------------Introversion (I)

How do you prefer to take in information?
(S) Sensing------------------I------------------iNtuition (N)

How do you prefer to make decisions?
(T) Thinking------------------I------------------Feeling (F)

What mode do you prefer for engaging the outer world?
(J) Judging------------------I------------------Perceiving (P)

able and takes little thought or concentration.

Now write your name with your non-preferred hand.

————————————

Notice the difference? How did it feel? Most people say writing with their non-preferred hand feels awkward, clumsy, uncomfortable, unnatural, slow, or sloppy. And it takes considerable concentration and time. You can do the job with either hand, but you're more comfortable using the preferred hand over the non-preferred one. The same principle governs the dichotomies. All of us function within the sixteen modes from time to time, but our MBTI code identifies those modes in which we are most comfortable.

YOUR BEST FIT

The questionnaire that follows is offered as a quick method for determining type. It is not, however, a substitute for the actual instrument. If you would like to verify your personality type by completing the full MBTI questionnaire, please visit my Web site at www.the8colors.com. Or you can learn more about the MBTI instrument, published by Consulting Psychologist Press, at www.ccp.com.

To gain insight into what your own type might be, consider the questions below. Read both sets of descriptions and check off those that are most natural to you. Which would you prefer if "nothing were riding on it"? Now note which boxes have the most check marks in them and transfer this information to the spaces provided at the bottom of page 9. There are no right answers; remember that we make use of all aspects of these processes at one time or another.

Enjoy the exercise.

DISCOVER YOUR TYPE

1. Where is your natural source of energy?

   Extraversion: Extraverted energy calls individuals to the world of people, places, and things, sparking them to actively seek engagement and stimuli in the outer world.

   Introversion: Introverted energy is founded in the internal world of ideas, thoughts, and feelings, drawing these individuals to reflective and solitary activities in order to energize.

EXTRAVERSION	INTROVERSION
☐ Acts, speaks—then reflects	☐ Reflects—then acts, speaks
☐ Openly expresses thoughts	☐ Selectively expresses thoughts
☐ Feels restless during extended time alone	☐ Savors extended time alone
☐ Talks more than listens	☐ Listens more than talks
☐ Seeks a wide variety of people and experiences	☐ Prefers knowing a few people and things well
☐ Speaks faster, more spontaneously	☐ Speaks slower, more deliberately
☐ Readily initiates interactions with others	☐ Tends to be more self-contained
# E _____	# I _____

2. How do you prefer to take in information?

   Sensing: Those who prefer Sensing gather information primarily through direct observation. They rely on tangible data and specifics to inform their reality, they trust experience, and they take a practical approach to life.

   iNtuition: Those who prefer Intuition tend to have theoretical interests. They rely on their facility with patterns and abstractions to inform them. They gather information through interpretation and connections.

SENSING	iNTUITION
☐ Memory is rich in details of past events	☐ Memory emphasizes patterns and connections
☐ Believes facts speak for themselves	☐ Believes facts mostly illustrate principles
☐ Trusts more in actual experience	☐ Trusts more in insight
☐ Starts with facts, then forms the big picture	☐ Starts with the big picture, then finds the facts
☐ Drawn more to what is immediately practical	☐ Drawn more to models and concepts
☐ Prefers knowing the facts of a situation	☐ Prefers knowing possibilities of a situation
☐ Learns best step by step	☐ Learns best through the big picture
# S _____	# N _____

3. How do you prefer to make decisions?

   Thinking: Those who prefer Thinking come to conclusions by analyzing data in a detached fashion. Costs and benefits are factored in to provide the best outcome. Fairness and justice guide the decision process.

Feeling: Those who prefer Feeling make decisions through personal empathy and identification. They are most concerned with values and the impact their decisions have on people.

THINKING	FEELING
☐ First considers cause and effect	☐ First considers impact on people
☐ Weighs facts and data to make decisions	☐ Weighs values and feelings to make decisions
☐ Is naturally skeptical	☐ Is naturally trusting
☐ Believes disagreement leads to better outcomes	☐ Finds that disagreement is uncomfortable
☐ Is won over by logic	☐ Is won over by an appeal to values
☐ Seen as forthcoming and objective	☐ Seen as personal and heartfelt
☐ In a work group, first thinks about efficiency	☐ In a work group, first thinks about harmony
# T _____	# F _____

4. What mode do you prefer for engaging the outer world?

Judging: Those who prefer Judging prefer an organized and structured environment. "Making a list and checking it twice" helps them be at their best in order to achieve their goals. Lists guide them.

Perceiving: Those who prefer Perceiving relate to the outside world in a responsive, flexible, and adaptive manner—"going with the flow." They prefer to keep their options open, putting off decisions as long as possible. Lists are a reference.

JUDGING	PERCEIVING
☐ Completes one project before starting another	☐ Enjoys juggling multiple projects at once
☐ Believes planning creates opportunities	☐ Believes adapting creates opportunities
☐ Seeks closure	☐ Wants more information
☐ Prefers sticking to the schedule	☐ Welcomes improvisation
☐ Separates work from play	☐ Enjoys mixing work and play
☐ Finds that routine is comfortable	☐ Finds that flexibility is comfortable
☐ Likes to have things settled	☐ Is excited by spontaneity
# J _____	# P _____

Below, circle the letter with the most check marks in each category.

YOUR BEST FIT

E or I   S or N   T or F   J or P

Keep in mind that this is an indication of your type. There are always factors in play that might incline you to respond to a description in a way that could create a false result. As you read this book, if your best fit type does not ring true, go back and review the questionnaire, paying special attention to the close scores. Choose the opposite description and see if that type fits better. Have fun discovering your best fit and exercise personality!

DELVING DEEPER INTO TYPE DYNAMICS

Some of the remarkable success of the MBTI system is derived from the fact that benefits can be reaped immediately from an initial understanding of just one preference. For instance, I've had people tell me that understanding there was such a thing as Introversion—and that it's a perfectly okay way to be—was itself a life-changing realization.

Each individual has a dominant and an auxiliary preference. A dominant preference is at the core of the personality; the auxiliary preference balances it. If a dominant preference is a Judging function, the auxiliary is a Perceiving function, and vice versa.

But there is more to the MBTI than eight preferences. As stated earlier, these eight combine in various forms to create a total of sixteen distinct personality types. To understand your type code to its fullest advantage, then, a little more should be understood about the way the preferences function together.

Sensing: There are two expressions of Sensing, and, although they both gather information in the form of facts and data through experience of the senses, they diverge in some particulars.

Introverted Sensing (Si) observes the present, but quickly reflects on the past for verification and comparison. The present triggers vivid memories of past experiences. Those with this preference are traditional in their choices and gravitate to strategies that have proven effective in the past.

Extraverted Sensing (Se) exists in the present, naturally taking in concrete data and the specifics of the physical world. Those with this preference have excellent navigational skills and enjoy observing and responding to the physical world in real time.

Intuition: The two kinds of Intuition deal in general with patterns and abstractions, but diverge in particular ways.

Introverted Intuition (Ni) receives and connects patterns and abstractions internally. New ideas and possibilities rise to consciousness most often during time alone. Those with the Ni preference are attracted to routine, which frees their minds to enter a "zone" that allows for

Whatever the circumstances of your life, whatever your personal ties, work, and responsibilities, the understanding of type can make your perceptions clearer, your judgments sounder, and your life closer to your heart's desire.

—Isabel Myers, *Gifts Differing* (1980)

innovative thoughts to emerge from within.

Extraverted Intuition (Ne) naturally and seamlessly connects ideas and possibilities in the external world. Those with an Ne preference enjoy opportunities to make connections and to engage the world of ideas and possibilities.

Thinking: Both expressions of Thinking tend to take an impersonal and skeptical approach to decision making, accepting cause-and-effect reasoning, yet they differ in particular ways.

Introverted Thinking (Ti) makes decisions using a subjective process of logical analysis and evaluation, measuring new perceptions against an existing internal framework.

Extraverted Thinking (Te) seeks to identify categories, or principles, and rules of logic that can be observed, discussed, and agreed upon by others. People with this preference then seek to apply these stipulated rules and principles to reach judgments.

Feeling: Both types of Feeling judgments include a personal approach to decision-making and generally consider, at the outset, the impact of decisions on the people involved. Those with this preference often perceive agreements and disagreements as personal.

Introverted Feeling (Fi) begins the decision process by subjectively measuring and judging a situation against an existing set of values. Internal harmony is what guides their decision.

Extraverted Feeling (Fe) appears more warm and empathic and may be more visibly distressed by conflict. Extraverted Feelers make judgments based upon external harmony and socially appropriate norms.

These descriptions, and the structure of personality as indicated by MBTI type codes and the concepts they represent, may take a little time to digest. But keep in mind that they all refer to the basic four dimensions or dichotomies explained at the beginning of this chapter. Throughout the book, we'll continue to explore these terms and concepts to help you gain greater understanding of your type. In the next chapter, you'll discover how to translate type into The 8 Colors of Fitness program.

An understanding of type frees you in several ways. It gives you confidence in your own direction of development—the areas in which you can become excellent with the most ease and pleasure. It can also reduce the guilt many people feel at not being able to do everything in life equally well.
—Gordon Lawrence, *People Types & Tiger Stripes* (2000)

"THE SIXTEEN TYPES AT A GLANCE" by Charles R. Martin

ISTJ	ISTP	ISFP
For ISTJs the dominant quality in their lives is an abiding sense of responsibility for doing what needs to be done in the here-and-now. Their realism, organizing abilities, and command of the facts lead to their completing tasks thoroughly and with great attention to detail. Logical pragmatists at heart, ISTJs make decisions based on their experience and with an eye to efficiency in all things. ISTJs are intensely committed to people and to the organizations of which they are a part; they take their work seriously and believe others should do so as well.	For ISTPs the driving force in their lives is to understand how things and phenomena in the real world work so they can make the best and most effective use of them. ISTPs are logical and realistic people, and they are natural troubleshooters. When not actively solving a problem, ISTPs are quiet and analytical observers of their environment, and they naturally look for the underlying sense to any facts they have gathered. ISTPs do often pursue variety and even excitement in their hands-on experiences. Although they do have a spontaneous, even playful side, what people often first encounter with them is their detached pragmatism.	For ISFPs the dominant quality in their lives is a deep-felt caring for living things, combined with a quietly playful and sometimes adventurous approach to life and all its experiences. ISFPs typically show their caring in very practical ways, since they often prefer action to words. Their warmth and concern are generally not expressed openly, and what people often first encounter with ISFPs is their quiet adaptability, realism, and "free spirit" spontaneity.

ISFJ		INTP
For ISFJs the dominant quality in their lives is an abiding respect and sense of personal responsibility for doing what needs to be done in the here-and-now. Actions that are of practical help to others are of particular importance to ISFJs. Their realism, organizing abilities, and command of the facts lead to their thorough attention in completing tasks. ISFJs bring an aura of quiet warmth, caring, and dependability to all that they do; they take their work seriously and believe others should do so as well.		For INTPs the driving force in their lives is to understand whatever phenomenon is the focus of their attention. They want to make sense of the world -- as a concept -- and they often enjoy opportunities to be creative. INTPs are logical, analytical, and detached in their approach to the world; they naturally question and critique ideas and events as they strive for understanding. INTPs usually have little need to control the outer world, or to bring order to it, and they often appear very flexible and adaptable in their lifestyle.

INFJ	INFP	INTJ
For INFJs the dominant quality in their lives is their attention to the inner world of possibilities, ideas, and symbols. Knowing by way of insight is paramount for INFJs, and they often manifest a deep concern for people and relationships as well. INFJs often have deep interests in creative expression as well as issues of spirituality and human development. While the energy and attention of INFJs are naturally drawn to the inner world of ideas and insights, what people often first encounter with INFJs is their drive for closure and for the application of their ideas to people's concerns.	For INFPs the dominant quality in their lives is a deep-felt caring and idealism about people. They experience this intense caring most often in their relationships with others, but they may also experience it around ideas, projects, or any involvement they see as important. INFPs are often skilled communicators, and they are naturally drawn to ideas that embody a concern for human potential. INFPs live in the inner world of values and ideals, but what people often first encounter with the INFP in the outer world is their adaptability and concern for possibilities.	For INTJs the dominant force in their lives is their attention to the inner world of possibilities, symbols, abstractions, images, and thoughts. Insight in conjunction with logical analysis is the essence of their approach to the world; they think systemically. Ideas are the substance of life for INTJs and they have a driving need to understand, to know, and to demonstrate competence in their areas of interest. INTJs inherently trust their insights, and with their task-orientation will work intensely to make their visions into realities.

ESTP

For ESTPs the dominant quality in their lives is their enthusiastic attention to the outer world of hands-on and real-life experiences. ESTPs are excited by continuous involvement in new activities and in the pursuit of new challenges. ESTPs tend to be logical and analytical in their approach to life, and they have an acute sense of how objects, events, and people in the world work. ESTPs are typically energetic and adaptable realists, who prefer to experience and accept life rather than to judge or organize it.

ESTJ

For ESTJs the driving force in their lives is their need to analyze and bring into logical order the outer world of events, people, and things. ESTJs like to organize anything that comes into their domain, and they will work energetically to complete tasks so they can quickly move from one to the next. Sensing orients their thinking to current facts and realities, and thus gives their thinking a pragmatic quality. ESTJs take their responsibilities seriously and believe others should do so as well.

ESFP

For ESFPs the dominant quality in their lives is their enthusiastic attention to the outer world of hands-on and real-life experiences. ESFPs are excited by continuous involvement in new activities and new relationships. ESFPs also have a deep concern for people, and they show their caring in warm and pragmatic gestures of helping. ESFPs are typically energetic and adaptable realists, who prefer to experience and accept life rather than to judge or organize it.

ESFJ

For ESFJs the dominant quality in their lives is an active and intense caring about people and a strong desire to bring harmony into their relationships. ESFJs bring an aura of warmth to all that they do, and they naturally move into action to help others, to organize the world around them, and to get things done. Sensing orients their feeling to current facts and realities, and thus gives their feeling a hands-on pragmatic quality. ESFJs take their work seriously and believe others should as well.

ENFP

For ENFPs the dominant quality in their lives is their attention to the outer world of possibilities; they are excited by continuous involvement in anything new, whether it be new ideas, new people, or new activities. Though ENFPs thrive on what is possible and what is new, they also experience a deep concern for people as well. Thus, they are especially interested in possibilities for people. ENFPs are typically energetic, enthusiastic people who lead spontaneous and adaptable lives.

ENFJ

For ENFJs the dominant quality in their lives is an active and intense caring about people and a strong desire to bring harmony into their relationships. ENFJs are openly expressive and empathic people who bring an aura of warmth to all that they do. Intuition orients their feeling to the new and to the possible, thus ENFJs often enjoy working to manifest a humanitarian vision, or helping others develop their potential. ENFJs naturally and conscientiously move into action to care for others, to organize the world around them, and to get things done.

ENTP

For ENTPs the driving quality in their lives is their attention to the outer world of possibilities; they are excited by continuous involvement in anything new, whether it be new people, or new activities. They look for patterns and meaning in the world, and they often have a deep need to analyze, to understand, and to know the nature of things. ENTPs are typically energetic, enthusiastic people who lead spontaneous and adaptable lives.

ENTJ

For ENTJs the driving force in their lives is their need to analyze and bring into logical order the outer world of events, people, and things. ENTJs are natural leaders who build conceptual models that serve as plans for strategic action. Intuition orients their thinking to the future, and gives their thinking an abstract quality. ENTJs will actively pursue and direct others in the pursuit of goals they have set, and they prefer a world that is structured and organized.

From *Looking at Type®: The Fundamentals* by Charles R. Martin. Used by permission of the Center for Applications of Psychological Type, Inc.

CHAPTER 2

Introducing The 8 Colors of Fitness Program

"Yesterday, I planned to work in the garden," says Karen, a thirty-four-year-old veterinarian. "But a friend called—'Let's go kayaking!' So off we went to Lake Champlain, with our bikes and our dogs and our kayaks in tow. For me, there's no such thing as an exercise routine. I keep Rollerblades, a wet suit, dry clothing, and a wind shirt in my car. I'm always ready for action."

"I like exercise that can be measured, because I'm not doing it for pleasure," says Candy, a fifty-five-year-old reporter. "I go to the Y twice a week. I bike for fifteen minutes, do the stepper for thirty minutes, and lift weights between thirty and forty-five minutes. I prefer not to talk to anyone. When I lift, I record sets and repetitions. That lets me know that I'm sticking with my program. I like to see that I did what I said I would do."

"Exercise is about being as alive as I can possibly be," says John, a forty-seven-year-old psychologist. "Play is the most spiritual thing I can do. Walk, bike, jog. I would never go to an aerobics or Spinning class. I hate the idea of a drill sergeant yelling, 'Go! Go! Go! Push yourselves harder, harder!' No thanks to boot camp. Exercise has to be fun."

Three individuals, with three very different approaches to exercise. And unlike two-thirds of American adults, these three have remained physically active for years. How do they stay with it when so many others give up or don't even bother to start? What do they know that others don't?

Despite their varying approaches, these individuals recognize that staying active improves their physical and emotional well-being. Sedentary people know this, too. And yet, according to a 2006 report by the National Center for Health Statistics, 66 percent of American adults do not participate in any type of exercise. In addition, 35 percent of adults are overweight, and another 36 percent are obese. (Report highlights may be found at www.cdc.gov/nchs/data/hus/hus06.pdf#highlights.)

Apparently, knowing that regular physical activity is good for us isn't enough. The health consequences of a sedentary lifestyle are no secret, including conditions such as heart disease, diabetes, stroke, arthritis, breast cancer, pregnancy complications, infertility, and depression. But a majority of Americans (and a growing number of adults in other industrialized nations) continue to resist exercise.

This puzzling lack of connection between knowledge and action is well-documented. Yet popular magazines and fitness and medical professionals continue to advocate for exercise in the same ways: "Join a fitness center!" "Create a home gym!" "Find a friend to work out with!" Despite good intentions, those who espouse these well-worn tips are for the most part ignored. Could it be that the way exercise is promoted, as opposed to exercise itself, is the problem?

THE SIMPLE TRUTH

The one-size-fits-all approach adopted by fitness experts and medical professionals alike is made up of valid points. They attempt to motivate people by emphasizing measurable exercise benefits—pounds shed, inches lost, increased muscle tone and cardiovascular capacity—which are all accurate, but miss a simple truth: *Physical activity is an expression of personality, and some approaches are more suited to*

Physical activity and exercise are like vegetables: they come in all shapes, sizes and tastes, and just about all of them are good for you.

—Michael Roizen and Mehmet Oz, *YOU on a Diet* (2006)

some personality types than others.

This is the secret at the heart of Karen, Candy, and John's remarkable success with exercise—they remain motivated to participate because they choose physical activities consistent with their personality types. This book will help you to tap into that secret by understanding your own underlying preferences and motivations so you can make better decisions about your physical activity.

The research for The 8 Colors of Fitness program is based on hundreds of interviews and self-reported data, addressing common aspects of physical exercise including motivation, approach, focus, preferred environments, interpersonal connections, and preferred coaching styles. I used a questionnaire (see Fig. 2.1, below) designed in consultation with a professor of research methodology at the University of Vermont. My interview subjects' self-reported activity patterns were correlated with their MBTI responses, which resulted in the emergence of bold patterns.

In Chapter One, you learned about type theory and the MBTI instrument and saw that individual personalities vary in their preferences for engaging life and making choices. In The 8 Colors of Fitness program, these type principles naturally and logically assist

Fig. 2.1 Research Questionnaire

Describe a typical week of exercise.

Where do you exercise?

What aspect of the environment is important to you?

Do you exercise alone or with someone else (others)? Describe.

What motivates you to exercise? Describe the benefits.

What types of exercise, interactions, or environments turn you off?

What coaching styles work or don't work for you?

What advice would you give people of your type who do not exercise to help them exercise?

you in discovering your individual fitness personality, a discovery that will help you to create an active lifestyle you'll be more likely to sustain throughout your life. Remember that it is difficult for people to maintain an exercise program if they attempt to exercise in a way that is incompatible with their type. They are doomed from the start.

By understanding the type theory that underpins the system, and by identifying your own color type and learning more about it in the chapters to come, you will recognize why you gravitate to certain activities and situations, and you'll clearly see the way to a more satisfying and active lifestyle, with less stress and resistance.

RETHINKING COMMON ATTITUDES

To understand the difference between generic admonitions to exercise and the 8 Colors of Fitness program, consider two of the most common concepts related to exercise and physical pursuits:

Exercise as clinical prescription. Our culture often characterizes exercise in a clinical way—treadmills, sit-ups, crunches—losing sight of the reality that any physical activity that uses your body and burns calories can come under the heading of exercise. Lifting weights, running a mile, playing a pickup game of basketball, or romping with your kids all qualify. The good news is there is no single correct way to include exercise in your life, and adding a measure of enjoyable physical activity to each day is within reach of just about everyone.

Exercise buddies. Another common assumption is that people are more successful engaging in physical activity in the company of other people. People are often advised, therefore, to find an "exercise buddy" to help them maintain momentum in a program.

This advice is not necessarily helpful. Pursuits that qualify as recreation or social events may be activities of choice for some people, but when goal-directed exercise is needed—for instance, when training for a specific challenge, or exercising to strengthen individual muscles—people may be a distraction.

SIXTEEN TYPES, EIGHT COLORS

As described in Chapter One, The MBTI® system describes sixteen basic personality types. Yet my program is comprised of eight colors.

Based on my research, I found that exercise and physical activity choices are closely correlated with the Perceiving processes, Sensing and Intuition. That realization lead me to create the color groupings for The 8 Colors of Fitness program. These pairs each share the same Perceiving process. Because exercise and physical activity are ongoing behaviors, it makes sense that the more open-ended Perceiving process (as opposed to the conclusion-seeking Judging process) would play a heightened role in sorting these activity preferences. This is consistent with Isabel Myers' findings that our lifestyle is influenced the most by our Perceiving functions.

The 8 Colors of Fitness program took shape around the shared Perceiving processes in the following areas:

- Motivation
- Approach to exercise
- Focus and attention: the role of the mind
- Preferred environments
- Interpersonal connections
- Favorite activities
- Roadblocks and tips
- Trainers and health professionals

A CLOSER LOOK AT EXTRAVERSION AND INTROVERSION

"If you're an Extravert, you should exercise with other people—if you're an Introvert, exercise by yourself."

This advice sounds like a logical extension of type, but is anecdotal rather than evidence-based, and it doesn't give practical information or guidance about what is truly effective. The use of type in making exercise decisions must take other factors into account to be useful. I've learned, for example, that Extraverts feel pressure to be

I think that anyone who comes upon a Nautilus machine suddenly will agree with me that its prototype was clearly invented at some time in history when torture was considered a reasonable alternative to diplomacy.

—Anna Quindlen

social when in the company of other people, which works when playing team sports that value cooperation, but can be distracting when learning a routine that requires concentration. In turn, some Introverts enjoy exercising alongside others when those people are involved in similar pursuits, but though they often appreciate light banter, Introverts may prefer not to converse at length or work in tandem with others.

In the language of MBTI, then, the terms Extraversion and Introversion do not merely describe a straightforward preference for either groups or solitude. These words point also to the direction of energy flow for each of the functions. Let's consider Introverted Intuition (Ni) and Extraverted Intuition (Ne). Whereas the two functions share an involvement with the abstract world of ideas, patterns, and possibilities, Extraverted Intuition is stimulated by connecting with others, and Introverted Intuition receives visions from within—two quite different processes.

The same principle is at work for Sensing. Both Introverted Sensing (Si) and Extraverted Sensing (Se) obtain information through the senses in the present moment. But with Si types, within a nanosecond that data travels through a vast storehouse of memories to be processed for verification and meaning—"looks like," "sounds like," "reminds me of," and so forth. Not so for Se types—for them, it's all about "Now!"

Most of the exercise choices and behaviors I observed were related to a combination of these factors within a type, rather than to a single factor. For example, I discovered that the length of time one prefers to spend either alone or with others varies greatly between Extraverts and Introverts. When it comes to physical activity, about two hours is often the limit

---

Perception involves all the ways of becoming aware of things, people, happenings, or ideas. Judgment involves all the ways of coming to conclusions about what has been perceived. If people differ systematically in what they perceive and in how they reach conclusions, then it is only reasonable for them to differ correspondingly in their interests, reactions, values, motivations, and skills.

—Mary H. McCaulley, *MBTI Manual,* 3rd edition (1998)

for an Extravert. After biking, hiking, or kayaking for a couple of hours alone, for example, Extraverts start to feel edgy and seek contact with people.

By contrast, Introverts can savor an entire day outside on their own, enjoying an activity such as hiking, biking, kayaking, or windsurfing. As an Extravert myself, this knowledge helped me select a kayak— I realized I didn't need one with a large storage hatch because I wouldn't be out for very long!

Thus, simply referring to Introverts and Extraverts and the presence or absence of other people is too simplistic. For some Extraverts, quality interaction with one other person can provide the necessary personal contact they find so energizing. Introverts often develop a facility for creating their own intimate space within a large group. They might minimize conversation or eye contact, use music to screen out extraneous sounds, or employ their skill at focusing on the task to mask the presence of people nearby. For these reasons, The 8 Colors of Fitness program uses Jung/Myers process descriptors like Introverted Sensing or Extraverted Thinking, rather than simply referring to an individual as an Introvert or Extravert.

LINKING COLOR TO TYPE

Throughout the research process I became aware that certain attributes of each type pair reminded me of colors that resonated with the physical energy of the type. The color code evolved as an accessible format that could be used to identify with and refer to when seeking information about individual fitness personas.

Refer to the chart in Fig. 2.2. on page 23 to locate your type and its corresponding color.

EFFICIENCY AND HARMONY

In discussing the manner in which Thinking and Feeling preferences differ within a color, I've chosen to substitute the descriptive terms *Efficiency* and *Harmony* for the two poles of this dichotomy. I cheerily admit to this heresy for a number of reasons.

First, I've long been troubled by how difficult it is to explain in English how "Feeling" is a rational function. I understand that Jung identified both Thinking and Feeling as rational, and I've read authorities who suggest that the nuance of meaning is more clear in the original German. But during my research—

and following my own Ni moment—I began to use the terms *Efficiency* and *Harmony* in discussions and presentations, and the terms seemed to elicit a clearer understanding of how the two preferences function within their types.

Obviously, in exercise as in other realms of life, the preferences are not exclusive; an individual inclined toward Harmony ultimately develops a level of Efficiency, and vice versa. But the terms have been useful in classifying, explaining, and predicting behavior and preferences. Accordingly, I use them in this work.

When discussing the MBTI type code, referring to Thinking and Feeling makes sense, as the coded letters refer to those variables. The language of The 8 Colors of Fitness program, however, uses the new terms, as you'll see in the chapters that follow. For example, an INTP becomes a Saffron with Efficiency, and an ISFJ is a Blue with Harmony.

Efficiency

Those with a Thinking preference, Efficients, tend to approach goals and activities more impersonally than do the Harmonies, who have a preference for Feeling. Efficients are not antisocial—they readily relate to people, particularly if those people are helpful in achieving results in a task-oriented environment. And Efficients appreciate people who hold them accountable to standards, raise their performance level, and improve their competence. But when goals are involved, other people aren't as important as they are for Harmonies.

Efficients happily acknowledge the quality of the professionals they work with, after first taking the time to verify that the professionals are well trained and competent in their fields. With their preference for Thinking, Efficients are analytical, expressing a natural skepticism that doesn't accept a claim without data or experience to back it up. If experts cannot demonstrate

> *What people choose to do with their spare time can also provide useful clues about Extraversion and Introversion. But, as with occupations, the most important question is not what people do but how they do it.*
>
> —Paul Tieger and Barbara Barron-Tieger,
> *The Art of Speedreading People: How to Size People Up and Speak Their Language* (1998)

Fig. 2.2 The MBTI Types and Color Personalities

- *Blues* (ISTJ, ISFJ) are loyal, traditional, dependable, and straightforward. They are committed and conscientious; in other words, true blue.
- *Golds* (ESTJ, ESFJ) are traditional and conservative, trusting authority and proven methods. The conventional color of achievement and recognition, once the standard for our currency, Gold is the obvious choice to represent them.
- *Reds* (ESTP, ESFP) are quick responders with high energy. They're where the action is. Red is the color that wakes us up, tells us when to stop, and directs us to what to look at.
- *Greens* (ISTP, ISFP) are nature lovers who seek to quietly merge with the outdoors. What color but Green could better describe them?
- *Silvers* (ENTP, ENFP) are energized by new ideas and possibilities, ready to reset their sights to embrace novel concepts and opportunities. Silver is the color of mercury—shiny, fluid, and changeable.
- *Saffrons* (INTP, INFP) are strivers after clarity and seekers of truth. They're represented by Saffron, an out-of-the-ordinary burnt orange hue that commands attention but in a warm and comfortable way, without glitz or extravagance.
- *Whites* (INTJ, INFJ) are visionaries, with a connection to the unconscious that yields an endless stream of ideas and abstractions. A blank canvas exemplifies this type, pure white and receptive to the imagery of their creative mind.
- *Purples* (ENTJ, ENFJ) are quick of step, outgoing and self-assured. The color Purple matches their regal bearing.

knowledge and skill, an Efficient is unlikely to invest confidence in them.

When relating to people within the framework of a task, aside from observing basic courtesies, Efficients are logical and pragmatic. They are concerned with how well someone can assist them in achieving their goals. A well-run organization is expected to be courteous. Friendliness does not hook Efficients as it does Harmonies.

I noticed that Efficients seldom talked about the people involved in their exercise programs in a personal way. They didn't mention trainers at the gym by name and seldom mentioned a favorite coach. Any discussion of such people was purely functional: Are they good at what they do? Do they help the process along? Do they help achieve goals?

Efficients pay attention to the physical setup and availability of resources at a gym. Equipment needs to be accessible and in good condition. Their efficiency is expressed in a task-focused nature.

Karen, an ENTJ CEO—a Purple with Efficiency—is typical. "My objective is to work out six times a week," she says. Her focus on the "objective" is the language of a Thinking type.

"A good coach is someone who helps me maximize my potential, not someone who bullies me or tells me I'm great," Karen says. "I do love cycling with one other person. I wind up getting more benefits if I'm pushed." Again, hear the pragmatic language of an Efficient—focused on benefits, with people factored into the equation as a means to an end.

Skeptical by nature, Efficients rely on facts and data, seek expert advice, and challenge trainers to back up the information they provide. Golds (ESJ) and Blues (ISJ) especially trust credentialed experts. Silvers (ENP) and Saffrons (INP) respond to proven competence, logical explanations, and supporting data.

Harmony

On the other hand, as I interviewed individuals preferring Harmony (those with a Feeling preference), the overriding common denominator was their focus on the personal. This focus is influential in guiding them toward conditions and circumstances conducive to peaceful, harmonious environments. Harmonies value personal connections, holding trainers and teachers in high esteem.

Panio is an INFP, a Saffron with Harmony and a student of Tae Kwon Do.

He speaks of his study and his two teachers in unmistakable Harmony fashion: "They are remarkable, inspiring men," he says. "Both stress humility and self-awareness, cooperation and persistence, and the fundamental spirituality of martial arts. It was never about fighting and domination. It was always about self-mastery, about conquering fear and ego, and continuing to strive for perfection, the impossible goal." He says, too: "What I enjoyed, I found, was the sense of community—the cooperation—and to a lesser extent, the competition."

In some situations, Harmonies exercised choices that limited their need to interact with other people. A desire to maintain relationships was viewed as a hindrance when personal concerns thwarted their exercise intentions. For example, one Gold with Harmony (ESFJ) is uncomfortable being around people she can't interact with—or as she puts it, "complete an interaction with"—and thus prefers avoiding exercise classes altogether. A Purple with

Harmony (ENFJ)—even though a dominant Extravert—may prefer exercising alone to avoid accommodating a natural tendency to please others.

A corollary of this preference for establishing good relationships is the importance of physical surroundings. Typical comments from Harmonies emphasize atmosphere and ambience, perhaps noticing soft lighting and a pleasant view. Even when they structure their activity to avoid having to interact with or please others, Harmonies orient to people in the environment and like to have warm relationships with those they meet at their gym or in the neighborhood where they walk and bike.

MORE FACTORS TO CONSIDER

There are additional factors at work within each color. Remember, even though your own color code will be the most specific to you, you will likely share occasional aspects with other colors. You have a few of the

---

Describing an Si Manager: He is persevering, patient, works steadily with a realistic view of how long a task will take, seldom makes errors of fact, tends to be outstanding at precision work, and can be counted ont o follow through on commitments.

—David Kiersey and Marilyn Bates, *Please Understand Me* (1984)

letters in common, after all. As you learn more and gain a deeper understanding of type dynamics and all the fitness personalities, the prescriptives of The 8 Colors of Fitness program become even more personal.

Job or Pleasure?

Each of the eight colors and sixteen MBTI types enjoys a certain romance with their Perceiving functions, which exert a strong influence on exercise choices. Consider Extraverted Intuitives—Silvers (ENPs) and Saffrons (INPs)—who enjoy a chance to connect with new ideas and possibilities. Introverted Intuitives—Whites (INJs) and Purples (ENJs)—are intrigued by their internal visions. Introverted Sensors—Blues (ISJs) and Golds (ESJs)—are drawn in by recollection of memories.

For Extraverted Sensors—Reds (ESPs) and Greens (ISPs)—their romance is with the physical world of *now*. But while Reds are robust and at-the-ready, Greens merge with the physical world in a quiet, leave-no-footprints style. Each to his own.

We're always either taking in information or drawing conclusions and making decisions about that information—Perceiving or Judging. How might this fact relate to exercise preferences and the job-or-pleasure divide?

Early in the course of my research, I became aware that people talked about such factors as whether or not they were engaged by their activities and whether or not their exercise choices enabled distraction. Many respondents talked about exercise in terms of whether it required a level of attention, for example, or whether it allowed their minds to drift elsewhere. Conversations with subject after subject referenced how some exercises demand more attention to details and others offer opportunities to put the busy inner dialogue on hold and free the mind to muse on ideas or entertain visions. Sure enough, these differences divided along type patterns.

My husband is a Silver with Efficiency (ENTP), with dominant Extraverted Intuition and auxiliary Introverted Thinking. When he returns from a brisk walk alone, he often goes straight to the phone to attend to business. He's been out exercising in a way that

---

Walking is the best possible exercise. Habituate yourself to walk very far.

—Thomas Jefferson, 1743-1826

engages his Introverted Thinking, allowing him to make decisions, come to conclusions, and take action.

As a Purple with Harmony (ENFJ), with auxiliary Introverted Intuition and dominant Extraverted Feeling, I enjoy going for a solitary walk, a swim, or a bike ride. I return with insights. My first words are often, "I *just* had an idea!" Understanding this about myself now, I often intentionally go out for repetitious, brisk exercise "just to see what comes up."

For Saffrons (INTP, INFP), exercise is all about fun. Regular users of type might think of Saffrons as perfectionists, reserved and intense. Yet my research led to a different conclusion. When it came to exercise, Saffron after Saffron insisted: "It has to be fun;" "I just need to enjoy it;" "If it isn't fun, I'm not likely to do it;" and other variations on the theme.

I studied the interviews with other consistent exercisers and noted that some colors—notably Silvers (ENPs), Reds (ESPs), and Greens (ISPs)—also tended to follow the pleasure principle. Perhaps they weren't as single-minded and unequivocal as Saffrons, but unmistakably they were in the "gotta-have-fun" category, too. As a student and practitioner of the MBTI, I recognized the common denominator shared by the four colors. Each extraverted his or her Perceiving process; in the parlance of the MBTI, they were Ps.

What about the Js, I wondered? Did they share this need for fun so much on the mind of Extraverted Perceiving Ps? I thought back to one of my early articles on exercise and type that pre-dated the creation of The 8 Colors of Fitness program (*APT Bulletin*, Fall 2002). As I wrote then:

I interviewed the CEO of a local business. David is 40 years old, thin, handsome, and fit. He has preferences for ISTJ [Blue with Efficiency]. Prior to being at work in the morning, David exercises at a fitness center convenient to his office. He exercises five mornings a week, systematically rotating between cardiovascular and weights. He runs through the same program every week.

"Are you happy with your level of exercise?" was my final question in our interview.

David responded, "It gets the job done."

In the tradition of type dynamics, people like David have a preference for Extraverted Judging—in MBTI terminology, the Js.

For them, making the commitment and following through to completion are higher motivators than enjoyment.

I found consistently that not only the Blues (ISJs), but also the Golds (ESJs), Purples (ENJs), and Whites (INJs), didn't need their physical activity to be fun. In fact, they rarely mentioned fun when talking about their routines. That is not to say that they didn't enjoy themselves—quite often they found ways to exercise that were deeply satisfying, even spiritual at times— but fun wasn't what got them to initiate a fitness regimen and stay with it.

I began to see this element of pleasure on a continuum, ranging from enjoyment to fun to play. Js often found exercise pleasurable; it provided a sense of accomplishment and order to their day. Ps, on the other hand used the word "fun" all the time.

In fact, Ps found it more difficult to create a sustainable habit of exercise without some sort of "fun" connection. They wanted something closer to play from the outset, looking for enjoyment beyond the direct benefits of the activity itself. Taking a narrow view of what qualifies as "exercise" in our culture does them a particular disservice, and often adds a measure of guilt and discouragement when

they reject gym memberships or structured routines. The Ps I interviewed had conquered this obstacle and were often happily engaged in forms of exercise, such as sports, competitions, dance, and vigorous activities of daily living, that ably served their needs for both fitness and fun.

This has been one of the more interesting patterns arising from my research. Ps who attend my presentations on The 8 Colors of Fitness program often experience an astonishing "Aha" moment when I mention that Js never consider whether or not exercise will be fun. Needing that element of fun to get them past their own resistance, they're amazed that Js can sustain exercise programs they don't enjoy.

SHARED PERCEIVING PROCESSES: COLOR PAIRS

As I stated earlier, exercise and physical activity choices are closely correlated with the Perceiving variable. This correlation led me to create the eight color groupings for The 8 Colors of Fitness program. Within those color groupings, there are four related pairs based on their shared Perceiving function.

For instance, Blues (ISTJ, ISFJ) and Golds (ESTJ, ESFJ) share Introverted

Sensing, which is dominant for Blue and auxiliary for Gold. These types are conservative traditionalists; they have a concern for safety and respect authority and credentialed advice. Golds make a plan and dedicate themselves to accomplishing it. They're proud of their achievements and enjoy sharing their experiences with others. Blues are circumspect, careful, and methodical and prepare thoroughly for any project. When they make a plan, the commitment is primarily to themselves, and they're less likely to talk about it with others.

Reds (ESTP, ESFP) and Greens (ISTP, ISFP) share Extraverted Sensing, which is dominant for Red and auxiliary for Green. Both types are enlivened by outdoor activities, with Reds drawn to energetic play and robust experience and Greens to exploration and more reflective experience. Reds love a physical challenge and enjoy the company of others in competitive, vigorous sports such as in-line skating, racquetball, snowboarding, and basketball. Greens gravitate to solitary pursuits, such as long bike rides, river rafting, and windsurfing, spending time in the wilderness and on the water, where they can observe the changing seasons, notice new growth and signs of animal life, or watch the changing cloud formations overhead.

Silvers (ENTP, ENFP) and Saffrons (INTP, INFP) share Extraverted Intuition, dominant for Silver and auxiliary for Saffron. Both colors love the world of ideas and possibilities and a chance to make mental connections. They prefer activities with easy access and minimal process; convenience matters. For these mentally active types, exercise needs to be something more than just physical movement, or it's boring and too easy to put off. They like to be in flow, engaged by the activity, enjoying themselves. Once they begin something, Silvers are carried by the momentum of the activity. Saffrons become bored more easily.

Introverted Intuitives are the most intellectually independent of the types. They have a theory to explain everything, prefer innovative solutions to established ones, and are adept at seeing situations from an unusual perspective. Their skill at taking a very broad, long-range view of things contributes to their reputations as visionaries.

—Naomi Quenk, *Was That Really Me?* (2002)

They need to find an element of individual engagement—something playful that engages their fancy.

Whites (INTJ, INFJ) and Purples (ENTJ, ENFJ) share Introverted Intuition, dominant for White and auxiliary for Purple. Independent in nature, they share an affinity for planning and structure of their own design. Both enjoy repetitive activities, enabling them to free their attention during exercise to enter the "zone." Whites will avoid crowds, looking for a calming environment without too many surprises, allowing exercise to become a moving meditation. Both these Ni types think in categories: cardio, weights, and stretching. Purples will experiment from time to time, but are drawn to exercise they can make routine. They walk in the world with confidence and see exercise as a way to improve themselves, be more competent, and rise to the top of their game.

THE ENTRY POINT

The level of fun in an activity was critical for Extraverted Perceiving types. In contrast, the physical environment—whether a fitness center, swimming pool, spa, or yoga studio—was noticed acutely by Extraverted Judging types. They were "jarred" by things out of place or not maintained as they "should" be. Disorder prevented Js from relaxing and exercising effectively.

Knowledge of which side of the J/P divide you live on will inform your approach at the outset. For both Extraverted Judgers (Js) and Extraverted Perceivers (Ps), knowledge of type can clarify why certain situations loom like roadblocks before you can maintain a regular exercise program.

This may be better understood by considering some common characteristics of these type preferences. For instance, Js have a tendency to initiate, define/limit, and gain closure. By contrast, Ps prefer to respond, expand, and connect.

Ps work best when they can set their own pace and try out alternatives. If routines or schedules are too demanding, they may need a break to work on something else or at least an option to develop a routine. Anything that can transform the experience into something that's new or a little bit different will stimulate the P into increased productivity.

— Otto Kroeger, *Type Talk at Work* (2002)

By no means does my research indicate that, within the J/P divide, one side is more physically active than the other. I interviewed active and satisfied exercisers of all colors. What I found was that J's basic requirements are very real and very different from P's. It is in the nature of Js (Fe or Te) to orient toward routine, become satisfied with it, and, in many ways, take pleasure in the completion of their plan.

For the Ps (Se or Ne), the basic requirement is more often rooted in the interaction, connection, and the opportunity to turn their attention to the outer world. They need to notice and engage the environment outside themselves, whether the world of people, places, or ideas. These interactions provide the greatest satisfaction, which bodes well for initiating and sustaining an exercise program.

Remember Karen, Candy, and John from the beginning of this chapter? Applying The 8 Colors of Fitness model to their preferences, Karen's color type is Red, Candy's is Blue, and John's is Saffron. The 8 Colors of Fitness program will help you determine the workouts that complement your type, just as these active people did—the better to reap the rewards of a sustained, physically active lifestyle. In the next section you will be introduced to The 8 Colors and learn how fit and physically active people of each color naturally sustain an exercise program according to their unique personalities. Enjoy their stories as you uncover the hooks, patterns and preferences of each color.

SECTION TWO

The Colors

CHAPTER 3

ISJ, True Blue: Tried and True

ISTJ: Dominant Introverted Sensing with Auxiliary Extraverted Thinking
ISFJ: Dominant Introverted Sensing with Auxiliary Extraverted Feeling

Loyal, traditional, dependable, and straightforward: these are committed and conscientious people. In other words, they're True Blue.

There's a steadfast simplicity about Blues. With their modest nature, they avoid focusing attention on themselves, viewing such displays as boastful. Outwardly, they tend to underrate their abilities and accomplishments.

After other big picture types come up with a grand plan, Blues are the people who take care of details and implement it. If it's on the approved agenda, a Blue will go to work on it systematically, step-by-step, avoiding unnecessary sidetracks. Their execution is simple and no-nonsense, based on models and precedents.

They're economical in all things, including language. When you ask Blues a question, they answer concisely. They're not expansive and have never been accused of being long-winded. A typical e-mail from a Blue with Efficiency is short and to the point: "Yep," "Nope," "Here are the minutes," "End of year report attached." A Blue with Harmony might soften the language slightly, but Blues love the functionality and efficiency of computerized communication, which dovetails so well with their preference for conservation.

With Introverted Sensing as their dominant function, Blues naturally take in and store data. You can often see it in their eyes—they almost stare as they absorb the physical world

Books and articles are written about all the various strokes kayakers need to learn, yet I always ask myself, "What are the three most important points?" My motto is "Less is more."

—Scott, Blue with Harmony

and file it away in their internal data bank.

Paired with this tendency to observe and store information, Blues have excellent memories. They easily—some might say amazingly—recall past events in great detail. Their language is full of references to the past, verifying the present as it relates to prior experience. The name of a street walked down twenty-five years ago, what they (and you) ate for breakfast at a café two summers ago, the color of a kayak they rented on Lake Michigan, anniversary dates for friends and family—the past is as vivid to them as the present, neatly stored and easily retrieved. And I might add, they're a little baffled by what other types forget.

With a job in hand and specific instructions on how it should be done, Blues will quietly go at it, working behind the scenes, rarely drawn to action on the front lines. But don't interrupt them. They're quietly focused on what they're doing, never happier than when they know what's expected and can move forward to completion.

Ruby, a Blue with Harmony, volunteered to help with her granddaughter's campaign when Celia ran for state office, wanting to assist in any way she could. Celia, a Silver with Efficiency, had several hundred envelopes to be labeled for a mailing and, almost apologetically (thinking how boring it would be), she asked her grandmother to put the labels on. Pleased to be offered such a concrete job, Ruby happily accepted and quickly developed an efficient system to accomplish the task. Celia was amazed when her grandmother affixed all the labels in less than twenty minutes and reported that she was ready for her next assignment.

I asked Ruby if she had an example of the way she goes about getting a job done. Now retired, she'd been a second-grade teacher for forty years. A little embarrassed by having attention focused on herself, but willing to cooperate, she described one of her typical processes: "When I have a lot of phone calls to make, I first look up all the numbers in the phone book and write them down on my list. Once I have a complete list, I make all the calls."

For several years, Steve, a Blue with Efficiency, sat on the board of the Vermont Association for Psychological Type (www.vermontapt.org). When asked to take on the lead for a major event, he accepted, as long as he would receive the proper guidance on how events were run in the past. He was given clear instructions and deadlines, which he followed carefully, asking for help when he needed it. He made coordinating the event look easy.

As a follow-up Steve said, "There were a lot of details to stay on top of, but I was able to get information as I needed it the whole way through and found it wasn't so difficult." In a similar no-fuss way, Steve goes to the YMCA three or four days a week, where he has easy access to the treadmill and weight machines in a familiar and comfortable environment. Regular and routine exercise has been easy for him to accomplish for more than fifteen years. When I asked his advice for other ISJs, he said, "Set practical goals that you can report to yourself on."

You can often spot a Blue by their mode of dress: conservative and neat. Khakis and a blue shirt are a typical Blue man's uniform, with shirt tucked in, pants clean and pressed. Women have a Talbot's look—coordinated and conservative, not too flashy.

MOTIVATION, APPROACH, FOCUS

Physical activity for Blues must be safe and predictable. They look for a well-cared-for gym, equipment in good working order, and appropriate and familiar locations for running, biking, hiking, and swimming. These necessary elements allow them to complete an activity with less fear of injury or unexpected complications.

Internally motivated, Blues don't depend on external stimuli or the whims of the moment to exercise. They are not seduced away from exercise by more interesting things going on. Commitment to their word ranks high among the hooks for Blues, and they derive a significant level of satisfaction from following through on their plans. During her work week, Diane, a Blue with Efficiency, runs after work. She said planning has helped her make it a habit. "I pack my clothes the night before and include my inhaler for asthma. Doing this, I'm committed."

Blues are highly sensitized and aware of their bodies and thus are careful not to overdo it. They gravitate to traditional exercises based on proven methods, tested and trusted, the better to achieve their goals with a minimum of fuss or risk of injury. Because they are exercising for a purpose, it doesn't make sense to them to spend time experimenting on new routines. Why bother when they already know techniques that have worked in the past?

With little inclination to live on the cutting edge, they're not interested in the latest weight program being touted, or in getting their exercise in "fun" new ways like Zumba. Blues focus on the purpose of exercise. They'll have their fun some other time!

For instance, when Blues learn a free weight routine, they prefer to learn techniques for developing one muscle group to their satisfaction before moving on to the next. Once a technique is locked into their memory, they can comfortably move on, but not until. Correct form represents not only the best and least wasteful approach, but it ensures greater safety. For David, a Blue with Efficiency, safety just makes sense. "I avoid running outside at night and during slippery weather because I am afraid that I may fall and injure myself," he said. "Injuries are a huge inconvenience and interfere with my ability to exercise."

What you don't see behind their modest and quiet demeanor is what pre-occupies Blues' minds: data, details, facts, memories, steps, what's present, and what's missing. Knowing they prefer to exercise alone, I wanted to know what goes on in their mind that allows them to do basically the same routine day after day, month after month, and year after year. I found Blues were totally engrossed in the details of an activity and, for instance, were able to describe something as precise as a three-second rowing stroke in several pages of exquisite detail.

The best course in any physical endeavor for this type is to start slowly and master one aspect at a time. The Blue way is to set practical goals and practice correct form. Not only would incorrect form fail to achieve the desired result, but it also leads to injury.

Another signature strength of all Blues is their outstanding power of concentration. When they are working they can seem to be in another world, so intense is their focus. When they're in this state, interruptions are jarring and unwelcome. In the gym or out, with their goal in mind, they prefer to get it done and not interact with people.

Blues are motivated by keeping track of their workouts. What better way to measure progress and see that they accomplished what they set out to do than by writing it down and seeing the data in front of them? Record keeping allows Blues to refer to their progress in the orderly manner that resonates with their True Blue nature. Date, time, distance, exertion, set, reps, results— all details are documented.

Based on my informal observations, Blues are the most likely to use an "out of office" reply for their phones and e-mail messages. They clearly see the divisions in life, and they name them. When they're not available, they're *not available*. It isn't a good idea to call them on weekends with business questions that can wait. Work is work and leisure is leisure. Frequently in interviews, Blues made references to "weekend stuff": in other words stuff they really enjoy. They often remarked that the purpose of exercise is to be in shape for weekend stuff.

Many Blues enjoy a variety of sports, and you'll find them well represented in any gathering of talented athletes. As adults, many Blues prefer revisiting sports from their youth. But sport is considered different from exercise. They might use exercise to get in shape or stay in shape for their sport, but as noted, Blues don't demand or expect the exercise itself to be enjoyable. If it is, so much the better, but enjoyment is not the hook.

ENVIRONMENT AND PERSONAL CONNECTIONS

With an emphasis on safety and form, Blues value a chance to learn from qualified experts who can teach them step by step. Blues who join gyms look for convenient, safe places with the resources they need to accomplish their goals. They are not looking for extra stimu-

lation and view paying for amenities unrelated to their exercise goals as wasteful. Time-honored institutions hold special appeal, and it's no accident that many of the Blues I interviewed belong to the YMCA. They like comfort and familiarity and have no interest in moving to new facilities for the sake of change or novelty. Blues aren't bored with the "same old"; they are comforted by it. Blue-with-Harmony Sarah said it plainly: "When it comes to exercise, I'm not adventurous."

Blues seek calm environments that allow them to focus in on the task at hand. They find commotion and interruptions disturbing, so at the gym they will often use their iPod or a book on tape to help them create their own "quiet space" alongside others.

The outdoors is a favorite option, offering unlimited opportunities for quiet and contemplation. Blues observe the world around them, noticing animal tracks, seasonal growth, and changes. With a myriad of sensory impressions stored away, Blues return to their favorite places over and over to revisit these experiences.

I like running on the bike path because I can measure how far I'm going. I keep myself going by chanting a mantra. It takes my mind off being tired.

—Cathy, Blue with Efficiency

Blues' inward focus is distracted by cars, commerce, and city streets as exercise environments. They might even view them as dangerous and, instead, gravitate to areas designated for recreation—walking along a hiking trail or running on a bike path. They enjoy using their observational skills, maybe watching the loons and herons at a favorite pond. It's all good, alone or with a comfortable other.

Blues often exercise in the middle of the day, using this time alone to mull over concerns by themselves. "I like to exercise at noon," said Scott, a Blue with Harmony. "It creates the second half of my day. I debrief, process, get new energy. It's a critical part of my psychology and balance."

BLUES WITH EFFICIENCY (ISTJ)

With their serious demeanor and conserving nature, Blues with Efficiency are the ultimate no-nonsense types. Why say in three sentences what you can say in one—or better yet, why even comment at all? Conserving is the Blue with Efficiency modus operandi.

Their natural inclination to conserve prompts brevity in all things—instruction, conversation, memos, e-mails, feedback to others. It's not that Blues with Efficiency withhold information; to them, nothing more needs to be said. To expand would be an unnecessary waste of time and energy.

I took a personal strength-training session with Brian, a Blue with Efficiency, who illustrates this trait perfectly. As I worked on my bicep curls, Brian paid close attention, but said nothing. As a Purple with Harmony, I sought some feedback. "Is my form OK?" I asked. Brian said, "Suzanne, I'll let you know when your form is incorrect. Otherwise, assume it's correct." Now that's conserving!

Concrete and organized, a Blue with Efficiency's road to success leads to tangible objectives in an uncomplicated fashion. The more intricate the process, the more distracted and anxious Blues with Efficiency become. They want every aspect of their exercise program to serve a purpose, with no distractions, duplication, or frills.

"I am very pragmatic," said Michaela, a Blue with Efficiency who e-mailed me from the UK. "A suitable space and suitable equipment will do. Any equipment that is pointless, like those roller cages for abdominal work, or Swiss balls, makes me want to turn round and leave. As does touchy-feely stuff."

Traditional Blues enjoy yoga, but for

them the greater appeal is the flexibility gained from yoga practice, not the meditative aspect, and certainly not the spiritual readings that often accompany a class. So Blues, enjoy the stretch and forget the Namaste.

With clear goals and objectives and the requisite resources available, Blues with Efficiency enjoy working on their projects independently. And for them, exercise is just another project. A quiet gym with the basic equipment "does the job" just fine.

What happens if the place gets noisy? With their outstanding powers of concentration, Blues with Efficiency "tune out," which they do by "tuning in." You'll often see Blues with Efficiency exercising with reading material, or with iPods or books-on-tape playing into earphones. As one Blue with Efficiency said, "I can zone out and create my own space just about anywhere."

BLUES WITH HARMONY (ISFJ)

With a focus on hearth and home and traditional values, Blues with Harmony are hardworking, dutiful toward family and community, and well regarded for their contributions. They take their responsibilities seriously, and they're guided by strongly held values and dedication to loved ones and community. They quietly care for others, responding to their physical needs. Picture a Blue with Harmony preparing school lunches for their children after the little ones have gone to bed.

Blues with Harmony can be worriers. With Introverted Sensation, their vivid memories recall injury and danger from the past. Combined with Extraverted Feeling (auxiliary) this produces a desire to protect and care for those around them. Other types might see them as over-reacting to potential threats, but Blues with Harmony take a cautious approach, never jumping into new activities. They'll put their toes in the water first, then a foot, slowly gaining a sense of comfort and safety before taking the plunge. They project this tentative nature and concern for safety onto others.

With their preference for Feeling, Harmonies notice the personal; as Blues, they're highly responsible. Put the two together, and Blues with Harmony notice how other people handle their responsibilities. At a gym, they expect the people at the front desk and the other employees to be responsive and for the facility to be run in a welcoming manner. It's important to them that a gym feel like a friendly place.

With Feeling extraverted, Blues with

Harmony are concerned about their own proper behavior in the presence of others, too. Since they depend on the past to guide them, they can experience discomfort in new routines and unfamiliar environments where they're concerned about learning the protocol. For Blues with Harmony, variety is not the spice of life.

MEET THE BLUES

Candy, Blue with Efficiency (ISTJ)

Candy is a newspaper reporter widely respected for her precise research and attention to detail. Candy doesn't particularly enjoy exercising, but she's been religious about her routine for most of her adult life. She does it the Blue way—commit, plan, keep track, and stay with it.

For Blues who think of exercise as a job, part of the gratification is in knowing they've completed what they set out to do. And there's no better way than to measure their progress. As Candy notes, "I prefer exercise that can be measured because I'm not doing it for pleasure. I go to the Y twice a week. I bike for 15 minutes; do the Stair-Master for 30 minutes; and lift weights for 30 to 45 minutes. I prefer not speaking to anyone. When the weather's good, I run on the golf course. Because of work, I exercise at the end of the day, but I wish I could do it in the morning and get it over with."

All the Blue with Efficiency elements are there—a traditional and trusted location, a targeted program that's repeated from week to week, alone time, and no requirement for pleasure. Candy is exercising to stay in shape. She'd rather get it all over with early in the day, but she can't, so she honors her commitment to herself and goes in the afternoon. Candy is a True Blue.

"I always put in a program when I'm on the StairMaster," Candy says. "Then I have to finish the program whether I like it or not. Writing down and keeping track of my workouts is important. The Y provides a card to keep track of weigh-lifting workouts, and filling up the card lets me know I'm sticking with my program. I also record workouts on my calendar. I like to see that I've done what I said I would do."

Candy, with dominant Introverted Sensing, has outstanding powers of concentration and shows a significant preference for exercising alone. She frequently listens to books on tape and is discerning about her preferences for sound and topic. For her, it's English novels with a strong plot line, read in a British voice.

Like a true Blue with Efficiency, Candy separates exercise from other activities, carefully keeping exercise in the *work* category. "I love hiking, being outside in nature," she says. "That's one reason I work out, to stay in shape for outdoor activities, weekend stuff. I also love hiking because there's a goal—the top of the mountain. I always go to the top. I love being away from people, not being surrounded by people. I notice the plants, the foliage. I really notice the smells. I love the scents of the mountains, the balsams and ferns. I notice how the air feels. I love the cool air. When I retire, I want to be outside more."

Bob, Blue with Efficiency (ISTJ)

Bob is a computer consultant who also serves in the Navy Reserve. He lives outside of Washington, D.C., where he enjoys rowing on the C & O Canal. He is president of his boat club, and rowing is his mainstay exercise, a sport in which he competed during his college years. He no longer competes but now rows for exercise. "I prefer this to anything else," Bob says.

All of the traditional aspects of the boathouse hold appeal for Bob. "It's an old building," he says. "The entire interior is finished wood. It has a traditional feel—part of something that has gone on for a long time."

Bob now enjoys rowing by himself; that way he says he can control the experience. If he wants to work hard, he does; if not, it is up to him. He describes the physical environment as part of the motivation—a good environment that creates peace of mind, away from the city.

While rowing, Bob is engaged and focused on the precise execution of each stroke. He explains, "Good execution reduces the energy you need to move fast through the water. It's a frictionless exercise; the river is like a track. It's important to always remind yourself of the proper form."

During a seminar I gave in the Washington area, Bob demonstrated and

---

Painstaking with details, individuals with the Introverted Sensation pattern care about getting things done on time and according to precise specifications. When carrying out tasks, they will not stop until satisfied all that could be done has been done. They are consistent and persistent doers.

—Roger Pearman and Sarah Albritton, *I'm Not Crazy, I'm Just not You* (1997)

described a rowing technique for the participants. Later, he sent me a written description of the stroke. When I received three pages of detailed explanation to describe a three-second rowing stroke, I saw a True Blue with Efficiency in action. His description was a clear example of the level of detail that dominant Introverted Sensing is naturally drawn to.

Eric, Blue with Harmony (ISFJ)

Eric serves as Director of the Counseling Program at a large university, in addition to maintaining his own private counseling practice. Early in the course of my research, we made an appointment to meet for our interview at a bakery cafe where we could talk over coffee. Eric arrived, surprisingly a few minutes late. He was apologetic, telling me he'd been visiting his sister at a nearby hospital. I certainly would have understood if he cancelled his appointment, but honoring a commitment is an important value for Eric, and he hadn't thought to cancel.

Eric is another Blue who talked of exercise and the YMCA. "I belong to the Y because it's user friendly, and it reflects the best of the city's diversity," he said. "I like that it's a community place, with members ranging from families to old people, young people, singles, couples, and gay people. It is a bit tattered and worn, but it's clean and the staff is warm and friendly and responsive to complaints. I belonged to a private fitness club for fifteen years, but it wasn't well kept, and the staff was unresponsive to complaints. In addition, I didn't enjoy the conversations in the gym and locker room— too much macho and old-boy."

I asked him what a typical week of exercise is like. True to type, he gave me a very detailed explanation. "I exercise a total of eleven to twelve hours a week, three times during the week and twice on weekends," he said. "I do twenty to twenty-five minutes of cardiovascular, plus stretching, sit-ups, and push-ups. In addition, I walk when I can."

Eric uses the same cardiovascular machines each time he visits the Y. "It feels good to do the same thing," he said. "It's hard to change. I take comfort in the routine."

While he's aware of the other people who frequent the gym, Eric doesn't go there to visit with people. "When I work out I'm not very social," he said. "I do my own thing."

Jan, Blue with Harmony (ISFJ)

Jan is CEO of a wind energy company. At age forty-eight, she's thin, well conditioned, and fit. But she hasn't always been that way. Jan recently lost sixty pounds through a hospital-based weight-loss program that included exercise as a component.

True to type, Jan began her weight-loss program after observing the success of someone who went before her. "I never would have done this if it hadn't been for John," she said. John is an engineer at her company and a close friend who lost eighty pounds on the same program.

"My husband said he was going to do it," Jan said. "I'd gained a few pounds over the years, but I figured I would lose them on my own time. I've never been interested in fad diets and weight loss. But he signed up and said, 'Now it's your turn.' "

She followed the lead of her husband and her friend, but Jan said she "freaked out" once she signed up.

"Why was that?" I asked.

"Because there was no way in the world that I was going to sign up and not succeed," she answered. "I was not going to be part of the group and talk about getting there—reaching a goal—and not be successful. The instructor was going to tell us how to succeed, and I was going to succeed."

The weight loss program is offered through an area medical center—an environment that lends legitimacy and authority to the program. This is an important consideration for Blues, who value authority and expert qualifications. Credentials are a must. As Jan said, "It was research-based at the medical center—common sense plus good science."

The program built gradually and engaged Jan's preference for focusing on details and keeping track. "We were given a formula and asked to track a thousand calories of expended energy for the first week," she said. Jan enjoyed monitoring her success, using read-outs on the StairMaster to measure calories burned.

After a while, the instructor explained how to convert outdoor walking to a measure of expended calories. Jan made good use of the information. "I would walk seventeen-minute miles and call that one hundred calories," she said.

Jan has maintained her ideal weight for over a year. Walking is now her mainstay activity—she prefers outdoors, weather permitting. Sometimes she bikes, keeping herself going up hills by counting to herself. "Exercise outdoors provides two very important things to me," she said. "One is the chance to process stuff going on in my head and clear my thoughts. Sometimes I actually solve problems while walking. The other is the opportunity to see things—

changing leaves, wildlife, the sun and clouds—that gives me a great deal of pleasure and perspective. I actually crave it.

True to type, Jan seeks out quiet, safe routes. Comforted by familiar surroundings, she developed a repertoire of roads on which she bikes. "Quiet," she said. "Away from cars. Cars distract me out here in the country."

FAVORITE ACTIVITIES

Cardiovascular machines: Treadmills, elliptical machines, and rowing machines allow Blues to select a program and commit to it. Blues enjoy the ease with which they can record a workout summary and track their progress. They prefer using the same piece of equipment at each workout.

Rowing: Alone on the water, Blues are engaged by the synergy of rowing and its dependency on correct form. The tradition of the boathouse is also appealing.

Running: Blues prefer traveling familiar routes they can keep track of. When training for distance, they enjoy the readouts that some watches provide. When training for events, Blues follow established professional guidelines and prefer training by themselves.

Swimming and water sports: Swimming, sailing, canoeing, and kayaking are appealing to Blues, especially if they have grown up with experience on the water. Following correct safety procedures is important to ensure enjoyment.

Walking: A commonsense choice for Blues, walking is done on familiar paths and routes. They enjoy spending time with the smells and sounds of nature. Alone or with a friend or family member, they typically keep track with a pedometer—a favorite prop for Blues.

Weight training: Blues prefer to develop knowledge and skill, learning through a qualified trainer, before working out by themselves. They insist on keeping weight programs simple and straightforward.

ROADBLOCKS AND TIPS

Roadblocks:

- Safety concerns
- Other duties that take priority
- Over-stimulating or disorganized environment
- Disruption of routine or plan

Top 10 Tips:

1. Take steps to ensure safety and avoid injury. Check equipment, and review techniques and routines with professionals. Don't run at night without reflectors.

2. Gather information from authorities to establish the importance of physical activity.

3. Choose a gym or outdoor fitness site carefully, keeping in mind the need for calm and organization. Familiar paths and routes work best when exercising outdoors.

4. Make a commitment to yourself. This is a prime motivator for exercise.

5. Schedule exercise as an appointment, and put it on the list.

6. Track progress and maintain records, which are written reminders of commitments honored. Use Internet tracking sites and gym cards.

7. When learning new routines, build slowly, ensuring correct technique at each stage.

8. Keep exercise plans plain and simple; make them easy to execute to achieve your goals.

9. When traveling, investigate swimming pools, gyms, and walking routes ahead of time. Know hours of operation, rules, and pricing before you go.

10. Use your powers of concentration to create your own environment. iPods and books on tape help you tune out by tuning in.

BLUE WORDS

Commit, concentrate, correct, deliberate, details, document, dutiful, orderly, practical, proven, record, routine, safe, steadfast, straightforward, systematic

Blues at a Glance—True Blue: Tried and True

ISTJ: Blue Efficiency—Dominant Introverted Sensing with Auxiliary Extraverted Thinking

ISFJ: Blue Harmony—Dominant Introverted Sensing with Auxiliary Extraverted Feeling

Overall Qualities	Conscientious, committed, and concerned with safety, Blues approach exercise dutifully and without internal debate. They are highly attuned to their bodies and correct form is essential. Steady and methodical, Blues prefer to focus on one thing at a time. They enjoy keeping track of their progress and take comfort in following programs that have been tested and proven effective.
Motivation:	• Clear fitness goals and objectives • Keeping commitments to themselves • Accomplishing what they set out to do • Advice from health and medical professionals • Bettering performance in sports and other activities
Approach:	• Rely on safe and proven methods • Build their program slowly, step by step • Choose the most conservative approach to accomplishing their goals • Seek routine—little interest in variety

Focus:	• Correct form and proper technique • Highly sensitized body awareness • Measuring, monitoring, and recording activities • Maintain energy using repetitions, chanting, songs, mantras, etc., while engaged in cardio activities • Excellent concentration for reading or listening to books on tape while engaging in repetitious cardio activities
Environments:	• Prefer safe, calm, and traditional environments • Attracted to familiar and predictable surroundings • Able to create private space within larger environments (with headsets or reading) • Prefer to be in nature—away from commerce and distractions
Interpersonal Connections:	• Prefer solitary routine exercise, with minimal gym interactions • Responding to people is distracting and de-motivating • Alone outside, or with comfortable other
Sample Quotes:	*I like exercise that can be measured because I'm not doing it for pleasure. I go to the gym three times a week. I always record my sets and repetitions. That lets me know that I'm sticking to my program. I like to see that I did what I said I would do. I prefer not to talk to anyone.* *Blue Efficiency* *I exercise three times a week at the Y. I use the same cardiovascular machines each time. I take comfort in routine. I belong to the Y because it is user friendly and reflects the best of the city's diversity. The Y is clean, friendly, and the staff is responsive to complaints.* *Blue Harmony*

CHAPTER 4

ESJ, The Gold Standard: Just the Facts

ESTJ: Dominant Extraverted Thinking with Auxiliary Introverted Sensing
ESFJ: Dominant Extraverted Feeling with Auxiliary Introverted Sensing

Gold, the traditional color of achievement and recognition, is the sought-after medal, first prize in the Olympics. The Gold Standard is so dependable it was used it to establish the value of our currency. It's the obvious choice to represent ESTJs and ESFJs.

As mentioned in the Chapter Two, Gold and Blue form a color pair; they share Introverted Sensing, which is dominant for Blue and auxiliary for Gold, making them similar in many important respects. Both colors, for example, are conservative traditionalists who have a concern for safety and a respect for authority and credentialed advice. But each is also unique. While Blues are modest, with a penchant for behind-the-scenes settings, Golds enjoy sharing their accomplishments and don't mind the limelight.

The Nike slogan *Just Do It* sums up the guiding philosophy of these standard bearers among the color types. Golds decide, plan, set measurable goals, find necessary resources—

and then *Just Do It* (in contrast with Reds, to whom *Just Do It* indicates a spontaneous response). This is true in Gold's work, community, and family, so why not in exercise?

Golds seek a balanced life, aiming for moderation in all things. They're proud of what they do and seek measurable results. "Are there any other kind?" a Gold might ask.

Sensible, practical, responsible, and, most of all, task-oriented, Golds live by established codes and principles of right and wrong. They have a rulebook that guides their decisions: keep it simple, learn from the past, lead a balanced life, and don't forget to enjoy yourself.

Golds are friendly, outgoing, and curious about how others do things. They're filled with a reporter's questions—who, what, where, when, and how—and display an active interest in gathering the facts. Golds with Harmony enjoy connecting with others, including strangers. They easily strike up a conversation, naturally eliciting personal information.

Comfortable with the "traditional life," many Golds enjoy belonging to a country club. They take no issue with rules and dress codes, but rather are pleased to know what's expected.

Golds look to the past to help them plan for the future, believing experience is the best teacher. They value and trust rules and expectations of behavior. Golds believe there's a right and wrong way to go about everything.

Golds approach projects by breaking a job into smaller, manageable pieces that can be completed and checked off a list. Their motto is "Keep it simple." It helps them avoid being overwhelmed by the big picture or trying to connect parts before it is time. Their process is step by step, and they trust that approaches that served them in the past will lead to intended results in the present. As a Gold with Harmony told me: "I have set patterns that work for me, that continue to be successful today."

MOTIVATION, APPROACH, FOCUS

Golds' traditional and conservative approach to all things carries over to exercise; they avoid unproven, fad, or New Age methods.

To Marilee, a Gold with Efficiency, it's baffling why anyone would exercise in a way that hasn't been proven effective. She would see that as a waste of time.

When Golds decide to exercise, it's for a purpose—to achieve specific results. Once their activities are aligned with that purpose, they are carefully planned. That makes sense; like Blues, Golds are sensible.

Their motivation to exercise is typically rooted in information or advice from trusted friends, people they admire, medical or credentialed professionals, or past experience. Golds with Harmony often take celebrity advice to heart and might respond, for example, to celebrity trainers appearing on *Oprah*.

Al, a Gold with Efficiency, described his experience. "Until the age of forty-two, I didn't have the sense that exercise on a regular basis was important. I had friends who encouraged me—good friends, trusted friends. And they were in great shape; I could see they were better off from running. I read articles about the benefits of regular exercise in *Newsweek, The New Yorker, Bon Appetit,* and *The Atlantic Monthly,* and I became convinced of the benefits."

When these *Just Do It* folks have a purpose, the planning begins. As Sarah, a Gold with Efficiency graduate student, explained:

"I have to plan exercise and schedule it—particularly now that I'm back in school full time. My week starts on Sunday and goes from Sunday to Saturday. I write it down in a day planner. It helps me be more at ease when I know I've planned for it. Planning helps me have a base of fitness to which I can add on."

But before they embark on their plan, Golds attend to their primary consideration: safety. No aspect of exercise's benefit or practice will get their attention unless they're content that the safety aspect is covered. And following the rules goes hand in hand with being safe: swim with a buddy, don't stand in the boat, get everyone a life vest. Golds see themselves as the protectors of our society. In fact, Superman was probably a Gold—ever vigilant and attentive to the safety needs of the citizens of Metropolis.

Golds carefully note the presence of danger in the environment and are vigilant in protecting themselves and others from unnecessary injury. That means knives stored in a knife block, a rubber mat in the shower, and no sharp edges or dangling cords.

Whether for a marathon, bike race, or triathlon, when Golds train for an event, they rely on specific and established guidelines. They devise a training schedule that they will adhere to, but stop if they experience pain or feel they are overdoing it. They might occasionally train with others, but prefer to be alone, following their plan.

What sustains this type, enabling them to exercise year after year, most days of the week? This question was paramount as I conducted my interviews. Peter, a Gold with Efficiency, told me his mind had to be engaged: "I put myself in a trance. I daydream. I frequently fantasize that I'm a pitcher for the Boston Red Sox. Sometimes I pretend I'm a stand-up comedian," he said. He went on to describe a round of *Who's on First?*

Peter combines running and walking for up to two hours at a time, keeping himself entertained along the way. When he reaches

Decide in advance what you are going to do and for how long, then plan to exercise on that schedule for at least a month. Decide that missing an exercise period is not an option. Find a time, set a goal, and just do it.

—Janna, Gold with Efficiency

home, he rewards himself with a carefully measured sixteen-ounce glass of cold orange juice.

Matt, too, has an inner conversation going during exercise. A fit eighty-year-old and a gym regular, this Gold with Efficiency works out on three cardio machines for twenty minutes each, totaling an hour of cardiovascular time. I asked Matt what engages him when he's working out. "All the old show tunes," he said with a laugh. "I know all the words and I sing them to myself when I'm on the treadmill, the elliptical, or the rowing machine." He listed some of his favorite composers—Jerome Kern, George M. Cohan, Rogers and Hammerstein. "They keep me going," he said.

ENVIRONMENT AND PERSONAL CONNECTIONS

Golds are comfortable with predictable environments, where they know what to expect and what's expected of them. Fitness clubs, for instance, have clear rules of operation and standards of decorum. But with their close attention to detail, Golds aren't satisfied with just any club. It must be bright, clean, organized, and safe. Once they develop their favorite routes for walking, for example,

they might not exercise while traveling. The comfort of familiarity is gone, and the exercise routine goes with it.

Golds like a place for everything and everything in its place. Disarray is distracting and overwhelms their senses. Having too many things to pay attention to creates discomfort. Some Golds report that while on cardio machines they'll mute the sound on their TV. Reading the closed-captions is fine, but listening to and watching a program imposes too much stimulation.

Golds enjoy sporting activities, such as golf or tennis, that they can play with friends or couples. They were likely part of a team when they were younger and still consider activity with others appealing. Because Golds look for the right thing to do, they appreciate the structure and order of team sports and happily sign up. Rather than questioning it, Golds appreciate authority. They tend to accept established cultural conventions and are happy to follow along. You won't find a "Question Authority" bumper sticker on a Gold's car.

Golds with Efficiency are straightforward, optimistic people who don't like to be around complainers. They look for a positive environment. For Golds with Harmony, the emphasis is on finding a friendly, harmonious environment, and they have a hard time relaxing without it. They place a high level of importance on being greeted at the gym by the same people each time and prefer attendants who know them and address them by name.

At times, though, interaction is incompatible with getting the job of exercise done. With Extraverted Feeling as their first function, Golds with Harmony have a highly developed point-of-view about how they want to be with others, and they enjoy meeting, greeting, and hosting. But sweating alongside others in group fitness classes is typically not their idea of enjoyment. It doesn't enable an opportunity to "connect" the way they would like to. That's why Ann doesn't enjoy group exercise. "I see all these people and I don't have a chance to interact with them. That bothers me."

Though Golds enjoy mixing a bit of social activity into their exercise routine—and want an upbeat environment—they nevertheless make the purpose of the activity clear. Natural planners who enjoy ticking activities off their list, Golds are irritated if they frame an exercise one way and it turns out another. However, it's very pleasurable for Golds to enjoy physical activities such as hockey and soccer with others, as long as they maintain the distinction between exercise and socializing.

Betty, a Gold with Efficiency, considers climbing to be a social pursuit. With that understood, she's comfortable with whatever pace her group establishes. She also enjoys running with others—but she's clear about the benefits the activity is expected to provide.

GOLDS WITH EFFICIENCY (ESTJ)

Golds with Efficiency are natural planners who accomplish results by breaking tasks down into manageable parts. So natural is their sensible, practical, and matter-of-fact approach, they are baffled when they see other people tripping up their lives through lack of planning and not being sensible. They are attracted to plain-spoken English, and common-sense mottos are often posted in their homes and workspaces. "If it ain't broke, don't fix it," "Keep it simple," and "Learn from the past" are maxims embraced by this type.

Golds with Efficiency enjoy problem solving and believe that problems can be resolved by "expertly applying and adapting past experiences," to use Isabel Myers' description of ESTJs in *Gifts Differing* (p. 95). They focus on finding the resources to handle a problem and become frustrated when personal feelings interfere with a solution. With their dominant Thinking function, they are uncomfortable when conversations get too personal. When this happens, they become bored and quickly steer the conversation back to more manageable language with a focus on applying resources toward a solution.

Golds with Efficiency thrive on a balanced and sensible life. They naturally conserve their energy and are aware of and responsive to their bodies. This inclination toward conservation frequently leads Golds to fit exercise into an existing routine. "I work exercise into the normal routine as much as possible so it doesn't feel like exercise," said Marilee. "During the workday, I walk to meetings at different sites. I take the stairs instead of the elevator. I don't enjoy exercise when that's all I'm doing. I see that as just another task."

Jon, a Gold with Efficiency, enthusiastically describes how he and his wife fit their forty-five-minute walk in between school bus pick-ups for their two sons. It's a practical plan and an efficient use of time.

GOLDS WITH HARMONY (ESFJ)

While Golds with Efficiency have a robust friendliness, Golds with Harmony are warm. They easily meet and connect with others on a personal level and have no problem striking up conversations with complete strangers. You can rely on them to hold up more than their share of the conversation. In fact, it's unnatural and unsettling for them to proceed in a relationship without first establishing a personal connection.

With Extraverted Feeling coupled with Introverted Sensing, Golds with Harmony are natural gatherers of personal information. In doing so, they display a disarming warmth and knack for putting others at ease. When they ask, "What's going on?" they really want to know. Feedback is fundamental for these information seekers. In fact,

I walk on the treadmill every morning for forty-five minutes. I plan most of my life, including exercise. I preset in my mind what I need to do. I even put out my clothes the night before.

—Susan, Gold with Efficiency

when they are unable to connect and get the personal information and feedback they need, they're uncomfortable. This discomfort can quickly turn to criticism of the circumstances, and they'll look for an exit. For Golds with Harmony, trainer feedback and friendliness are a must!

Golds with Harmony notice and want to be noticed by others. They enjoy routines that connect them to others and enable them to see the same people frequently. For instance, eighty-five-year-old Germaine has walked up and down the sidewalks on the same neat street in Cambridge, Massachusetts, for nearly a half a century. She walks year round, even through the cold winter. She knows her neighbors and they know her. She enjoys the friendly waves and the familiar environment on her two-mile walk.

MEET THE GOLDS

Deb, Gold with Efficiency (ESTJ)

Deb began exercising twenty years ago and has modified her routine little since then. "What motivates you to exercise?" I asked.

Deb answered immediately, "I want definition in my limbs." She went on to describe how she started. "Initially I was motivated to exercise after the birth of my two children.

I wanted my body back. I began working on muscle definition in my arms and legs. At five feet, ten inches and a 129 pounds, I'm tall, with long legs. It's not attractive to be bony. My weight hasn't changed in twenty years, but now I have definition in my arms, legs, butt, glutes—it's visible. Every muscle group is toned."

Deb is in terrific shape, and I found it interesting that her exercise plan consists only of weight lifting—no cardio. "I find cardio boring," she said. "I have nothing to focus on. Twenty years ago, I consulted with a certified personal trainer who said weight training is enough as long as I do it at a cardio clip. So I weight train at a cardio rate—I keep a steady pace. Once I get going, I don't stop. I don't let my muscles cool off."

"When I'm lifting I can count the sets, the reps—I'm keeping track of things. I feel my muscles work. I enjoy the focus and awareness. That way I know I'm working. I feel my chest, my back. and I know I'm working."

Deb has little interest in altering a successful program that has done the job for so many years. Although her home is outfitted with weight training equipment similar to the machines at the gym, attempts to transfer her program to a home gym have never been successful.

"I like going to the gym—being around people but not interacting with them," Deb said. "That keeps me engaged." Deb enjoys the light camaraderie with the other members and with the staff, but this is not a social time for her—it's about getting the job done, reflective of her J approach.

Within the last year, Deb has added yoga to her fitness routine. "I learned about the history. It is a very old mental and spiritual practice. Not trendy—I'm not jumping on a bandwagon."

Deb is a good example of how people in each type can make activities their own. Many Intuitive types are attracted to yoga for the body/mind/spirit connection. Something as intangible as that doesn't provide the solid evidence of benefit and results that a Gold is looking for. As a Gold, Deb made her exercise decision based on a proven record of benefit. After researching the history of yoga, she was satisfied that sufficient evidence supported its benefits.

Arnold, Gold with Efficiency (ESTJ)

I drove to interview Arnold in his summer residence. His type was in evidence when he greeted me (and my car) upon arrival.

With precision and extensive hand motions, he signaled me exactly where to park before escorting me into his house.

Again, true to type, Arnold shared the stories of his physically active life with gusto and pride, sequentially and in detail. Unlike Blues, Golds love to share their accomplishments with others. Arnold's fitness story is about goals and their importance. As he said in our interview, you can't do anything without a goal.

At the age of seventy-three, Arnold is a fit and highly tuned athlete, but he hasn't always been that way. When he turned fifty, he was forty-five pounds heavier and rarely got any exercise other than walking.

At that time, Arnold was still working as marketing director for a large company in New Jersey. Around his fiftieth birthday, he signed up to run the New York City Marathon. As a Gold who appreciates authority and order, he set about preparing for the race according to established training recommendations put out by the New York Road Runners Club. He has since run the marathon five times, regularly finishing in the top ten percent of runners in his age group.

Arnold has marshaled his planning and time management skills around his fitness goals. "I'm a natural planner. I know how to prioritize my time," he said. "There's a way to go about training—break it down into pieces so you can see what you do. If I'm doing a century (100) mile ride, I first ride twenty-five miles, then another, and so on. If I'm running, I run for ten minutes, then another ten minutes, and so on—same with swimming."

With a natural ease and extensive gestures, Arnold described his training board. "I have a big piece of cardboard with 365 boxes—all arranged into weeks and days. Each day, I know exactly what I'm going to do, and I check off what I did." For a Gold, making lists and keeping track assists in achieving goals. While Arnold's training board might be extreme, even for a Gold, his type finds they can more easily stick to a plan if it is physically structured.

At age sixty, Arnold took a year off to accomplish the following goals:

- Complete a century bike ride in each state
- Climb the highest peak in each state
- Run three miles in each state capitol
- Swim one mile at the YMCA in each state

In bullet-like fashion, he ticked off the elements that comprise proper exercise: learn how to eat right, maintain proper hydration, use equipment correctly, maintain equipment, warm up, cool down, and use proper body mechanics for each activity.

Arnold enjoys being a role model for others, which is natural for Golds as well as Blues, who prefer to learn from role models. He is an active member of his church community and serves as a board member for the National Senior Games Association. He competes on regional, national, and international levels in the Senior Games in biking and track-and-field, where he throws the javelin. At seventy-three, he enjoys the benefits of his superb level of fitness, taking special delight in biking and hiking with his children and grandchildren.

Dave, Gold with Harmony (ESFJ)

"I work out to stay in shape so I can be injury-free," Dave said. "I stretch for fifteen minutes every morning." In true Gold fashion, Dave is focused on safety and avoiding injury. As he says, "The key ingredient in staying injury-free is flexibility."

Dave works out on cardio machines most days of the week. He maintains his engagement by keeping track of the readouts, something he says "makes the time go by." "I switch around on five-minute segments," he said. "For instance, I'll spend five minutes watching the distance, five minutes watching the speed, and five minutes watching the calories. I make a game of it, and it keeps my mind on what would be trivial."

As a dominant Extraverted Feeling type, Dave likes seeing the same people each time he goes to the gym. "I've now gotten to know everyone at the gym, which is nice," he said. He particularly enjoys it when a few of his buddies are there. "We challenge each other and track it—for instance to see how many calories we can burn in an hour," he said. "Or how fast we can get to one thousand calories. It's fun making it into a game."

Typical of Golds, Dave enjoys other sporting activities, including biking, skiing, and particularly golf. With an eye on the personal, Dave described an additional benefit of golf: "I can figure a lot about someone when I play golf with him or her," he said. "I am familiar with the surroundings of that environment. There's a lot to learn being with different people in the same environment. If I spend four hours playing golf with someone, I learn how they handle adversity, how they act under pressure, how they win, how they lose, how social they are. Within the box of that day there's a lot to learn."

Iris, Gold with Harmony (ESFJ)

Iris is a professional jazz vocalist and a music booking agent living on the outskirts of Baltimore, Maryland. She goes to a gym near her home twice a week, and she said, "I hate every minute of it." She runs through her weight routine quickly—able to get in and out of the gym in less than forty minutes.

"How are you able to stick with your program?" I asked. She said her motivation and commitment probably were a result of her fear of developing osteoporosis. Exercise is important to combat the condition, and she made a commitment to herself to work at it. "It means a lot to me to follow through on what I promise," she said. "It makes me feel I am in control of my life— that I did what I said I was going to do." Following through on a commitment is a hook for Golds and Blues. When they make a commitment, most of the battle is won.

"The gym is a small, clean, and relatively personal space," Iris said. "And I see the same people each time I go. That helps." These are other hallmarks of Iris's type; Golds with Harmony seek a pleasing environment and enjoy the routine of seeing the same people.

"How do you stay engaged during those forty minutes?" I wanted to know.

"I think how good it will feel when I'm finished," she said. "I think that soon I'll be driving home. Sometimes when I am struggling with lateral pull downs, I think of Christopher Reeve and say to myself, Shut up and just do it." As previously noted, role models are important motivators for Golds.

What Iris actually enjoys and looks forward to are her yoga classes and the personal relationship she has with the teacher, Wendy. "Yoga tells me exactly where I am, where I'm weak, where I experience pain, where I'm loose, where I'm tight," Iris said. "I like to know where I am physically, and yoga tells me that."

Iris loves her yoga class, held in a church nestled in the woods of rural Maryland. Beautiful views of surrounding trees can be seen from most windows. The room is clean and large. Everyone has enough space, as the classroom is limited to ten participants. The instructor, Wendy, has become a friend.

"Does Wendy talk in class or include readings?" I asked.

"She cites fact-based information from authorities that document the physical benefits of yoga as it relates, for example, to heart rate or cholesterol," Iris said. "Her readings emphasize practical laws of the universe, none of the New Age stuff that really turns me off."

"What about the New Age message don't you like?" I asked.

"I hate the preachy stuff that tells you how to be a better person. To me that's personal, and I don't want to be preached to in a yoga class. Anyway, messages about world peace and love seem so abstract and unobtainable.

"Instead of learning how to be a better person, I like learning how to be better to myself. For instance, when Wendy tells the class to let go of thoughts, be kind to yourself, and not judge yourself—I like that. Sometimes it helps to let go of my thoughts by picturing myself letting go of a New York Stock Exchange ticker tape." Being guided through a meditation on letting go of one's thoughts is particularly appealing to Introverted Sensors like Iris, whose memory of past events is so vivid.

Iris described Wendy as being personable, knowledgeable, and caring. "She keeps an eye on everyone. She walks around the class and gently corrects your posture, giving personal feedback." These Harmony hooks—gentleness, watching out for everyone, personal feedback—keep Iris engaged.

FAVORITE ACTIVITIES

Cardiovascular equipment: Treadmills, ellipticals, and stationary bikes are appealing to Golds. They track their progress through the readouts, measuring time, calories, and intensity, keeping their minds focused. Many Golds have a piece of cardio equipment at home that they use religiously.

Golf and Tennis: Golds enjoy these activities that have established rules of etiquette and engagement. They want to have a respectable game and will train for it with other forms of exercise. They improve their fitness so they can play better.

Running: Golds appreciate familiar outdoor settings where they can take in the details of nature and savor familiar sensory experiences on the same route. They typically decide in advance if they will measure a workout in time or distance and are careful not to overdo it, stopping if they experience pain or discomfort. A wise and common-sense approach means correct form is essential, and they will learn that from an expert or other reliable source.

Swimming: A favorite activity for Golds, swimming combines all the important elements—correct form, opportunity to experience their muscles, measurement, orderly lanes, and structure. In addition, they enjoy the feel of the water. Golds swim for a purpose rather than for relaxation or to "puddle around." Golds with Efficiency frequently are or were lifeguards.

Walking: Golds walk with purpose—either at a fast and measurable rate for exercise or with a friend or family member for a social connection. Again, being outdoors enables Golds to experience nature.

Yoga: Golds are attracted to yoga for the results—a stronger, more flexible body—and especially enjoy it in later life as a way to round out other physical activities. Golds appreciate yoga's concentration on specific muscle groups, and they respect its tradition and trust its history. They find it calming and appreciate the emphasis on "letting go of thoughts."

ROADBLOCKS AND TIPS

Roadblocks

- Concerns about safety
- Not having specific goals
- Not scheduling exercise
- Disruption of routine

Top 10 Tips

1. Attend to and satisfy your need to be safe and injury-free. Find a trusted trainer or coach who knows body mechanics and will set up a conservative program to assure safety.

2. Make a commitment to yourself and to others. Doing what you said you would do is an important motivator, and being true to these commitments is as important as exercising itself.

3. Share accomplishments with others. Part of the satisfaction is telling others of your progress.

4. Be clear about the goals you are striving for; for instance, exercise for the purposes of increased mobility and injury-prevention. Goals such as these make other activities you enjoy—such as golf, tennis, and skiing—safer.

5. Exercise at the same time every day, measuring time and distance and keeping track of results.

6. Keep the mind engaged during workouts by counting, singing, thumping, reciting, focusing on muscles, or manipulating with readouts.

7. Break larger goals down into smaller parts. Set a plan for each workout so you can enjoy the satisfaction of accomplishing it.

8. Chose activities that are tried and true and promise the results you're after.

9. Reward yourself for a job well done. You deserve a favorite treat or a shopping trip.

10. Develop a Plan B so when the pool closes, your treadmill breaks, or your walking buddy relocates, you'll keep moving.

GOLD WORDS

Authority, comfort, correct, familiar, focus, goal, history, measure, memory, organize, plan, purpose, robust, safe, share (results), structure

Golds at a Glance—The Gold Standard: Just the Facts

ESTJ: Gold Efficiency—Dominant Extraverted Thinking with Auxiliary Introverted Sensing

ESFJ: Gold Harmony—Dominant Extraverted Feeling with Auxiliary Introverted Sensing

Overall Qualities	Traditional and conservative in their approach to exercise, Golds avoid unproven fads or New Age styles. With a comfort with and reverence for tradition, Golds seek a balanced life, aiming not to over-do, including with exercise. Golds prefer structure and routine, valuing experience, safety, proven methods, and authoritative information. Proud of what they do, results are what they're after.
Motivation:	• Exercise for a purpose, e.g. to address health concerns, prevent sports injury, lose weight • Exercise as the right thing to do • Keeping commitments—sharing accomplishments with others
Approach:	• Consult authoritative resources for plan • Set measurable goals, then break goals into smaller, manageable pieces • Prefer exercise be routine and structured • Ensure safety • Learn correct technique the "right way"—sensible • Develop familiarity with equipment, route, routine

Focus:	• Monitor, measure, and keep track of performance and progress • Concentrate on the physical, including muscle groups • Engage mind with active inner, monologs, mantras, songs, recitations • Watch television while engaged in repetitious cardio activities
Environments:	• Gym—open, well lit, clean, and organized • Positive and friendly atmosphere • Traditional and safe • Outdoors—familiar routes and routiness
Interpersonal Connections:	• Train alone or with others, as long as they can accomplish goal and it fits into their routine • Share accomplishments with friends and family • Enjoy organized sporting activities with others
Sample Quotes:	*I exercise for my health and because you're supposed to. From time to time I get bored with my routine and consult a trainer to change my weights. He is simple and straightforward. He shows me what the training is going to do for my body. He understands my goals and where I'm at.* Gold Efficiency *Yoga tells me exactly where I'm weak, where I'm strong, where I'm tight, and where I'm loose. Wendy, my teacher, has become a friend. Her readings emphasize the practical laws of the universe, none of the New Age stuff that really turns me off. The room is clean. Beautiful views of the surroundings can be seen from most windows.* Gold Harmony

CHAPTER 5

ESP, Roaring Red: Now!

ESTP: Dominant Extraverted Sensing with Auxiliary Introverted Thinking
ESFP: Dominant Extraverted Sensing with Auxiliary Introverted Feeling

The color Red is where the action is. It's an attention-getting, "look at me" color. Red wakes us up, tells us when to stop, and directs us to what we should look at. Full of energy, it's just the right color for this vibrant, animated, play-hard type.

The convertible was made for Reds. The roar of the engine as they speed down the open highway, wind in their hair, sun or moon overhead. There's something for almost every physical sense—to see, to feel, to hear, to smell, to touch—which is just the way Reds like it.

Uninhibited, Reds take a carefree approach to life. They crave action-packed environments with lots of play and stimulation. Their homes are often filled with toys and games—activities for "kids" of all ages. The Twister board is set up in the family room, the garage sports a basketball hoop, and the backyard volleyball net doesn't come down until October.

Even at work, Reds may keep a stash of games and puzzles on their desks—a yo-yo, a miniature pool table or croquet set, magnet art. The walls are filled with images of family and friends skiing, white-water rafting, boating, and enjoying other robust outdoor activities.

Reds grew up loving and responding to the excitement and stimulation of the physical life. Chances are they were the ultimate outdoor kid, climbing everything, playing with ropes, engaging in sports, and doing just about anything on a dare. My brother Ronny, a Red with Harmony, would make a few phone calls (there was no text messaging in the fifties) and almost without effort, a game was on at the baseball diamond behind the elementary school. Glove in hand, he would leave the house to return hours later, barely in time for dinner.

Reds are great in a crisis, able to quickly tap their full potential. Think Spiderman, as opposed to the quintessential Gold, Superman. Spiderman is filled with adrenalin, jumping, scaling, and swinging his way to the rescue.

Bill, an optometrist, described his son, a Red with Efficiency: "Matt was a handful as a kid," Bill said. "Something had to be in motion all the time. He was totally involved in sports. He played whatever sport was available. And he was very funny."

Matt's school years were tough for him. "He was very hands-on," Bill said. "And he tended to verbalize thoughts with no preliminary processing." But today, Matt is a Navy SEAL, a perfect career choice, notes his father: "He's highly skilled at what he does—jumping out of airplanes, firing weapons, breaking into buildings, and blowing up stuff." Bill said his son is a hard worker when accomplishing something important to him. "He'll go 24/7 for things that matter. But Matt is either *on* or *off.* There's a burst of activity followed by doing nothing. He's kind of like a lion—he's either sleeping or attacking something."

"Matt is in fantastic shape," Bill said, "but he's not an exerciser. If he had to do it on his own, he couldn't do it." Matthew is typical of Reds, who don't resonate with the word *exercise;* it connotes boredom, tedium, and suffering.

John, a Red with Harmony, agrees. "I'm an outside guy. It's boring to just stay in shape. I have to have a great end goal."

For Reds who live in the moment, anything is possible. With little concern for the future and no inhibitions from the past, Reds pride themselves in "going all out." They have little tolerance for long-range strategic planning and even less for theoretical or philosophical deliberations. After a while, such conversations, which they consider pointless and irrelevant, bore them. If discussions go on for too long, they may even create a diversion to stir things up. And then, at least, they have a fire to put out.

I always try to work out before any important event or meeting. I feel more perceptive, my timing is on, and I'm better at reading everyone in the room

—Ronny, Red with Harmony

MOTIVATION, APPROACH, FOCUS

Exercise for its own sake, without an end in sight, seems pointless and boring to this goal-oriented type. Training for an event and participating in high action sports, on the other hand, provide focus, motivation, and, of course, fun. For Reds, "be prepared" is not a simple admonition; it's a way of life. The trunk of their cars can look like a sports-equipment swap meet. They must have their gear at the ready to take advantage of any opportunity that might arise.

For Reds, the Nike slogan *Just Do It* describes their attraction to spontaneity. This means Reds will avoid anything that makes them feel bogged down; even the schedule of a sports league might feel confining. On the other hand, adding their name to a substitute list could be fun. Getting the call at eight o'clock, grabbing a racquet, and jumping into action is more appealing to this type than planning a weekly game. Of course just the opposite is true for Golds— the more planning, the better.

Hugh, a Red with Harmony, describes his style as "catch as catch can." He enjoys biking to work with his law partners and friends. "The day before a ride we decide to do it. It fits the way I operate," he said.

Being physically active is a lifestyle for Reds, and they can't get too much of it. Attracted to variety, they love being outside, on the court, on the track, or at the beach, and are drawn to activities that involve speed and thrills and that demand quick reflexes. With their jump-in-with-both-feet personalities, Reds seek activities that grab their attention and bring their senses to life, such as mountain biking, bike racing, and water and Alpine skiing. They also enjoy fast-paced games of basketball or racquetball.

They're hands-on people who enjoy frequent short-term victories and intermittent competitions that give them a goal to strive for. Reds find exercise in and of itself tedious. But reframing physical activity as "training," with its sense of purpose, works. "Training" to stay in shape

---

A great competitor will feel they never lost a game. They just ran out of time.

—Francis, Red with Harmony.

for a sport provides a focus that helps them push through an otherwise boring routine.

Hugh said boredom is his Achilles' heel, and indoor, repetitious, or routine exercise soon falls away. "I'm not good at exercise for exercise's sake," he said. "It has to be fun and with other people." He and his wife bought a stationary bike and he tried going to the gym. These attempts at routine exercise lasted only briefly. "I must convert it to some activity that's pleasurable, like snowboarding or basketball," he said.

Convenience is key for Reds, although in and of itself it is not a "hook." Minimal process and ease of access serve their preference for spontaneity and appeal to Reds' playful nature. "I would jump off a sailboat and swim three-quarters of a mile, but I'm bored in a swimming pool," said Karen, a Red with Harmony. A typical e-mail from a Red might extend an invitation to hike or kayak to dozens of friends and acquaintances. There's no need to RSVP; pressuring anyone to show up is not their style.

Reds focus on what they're doing at the moment, thinking of nothing else. Hugh described his time on the basketball court: "I don't zone out or get distracted by thinking about other things," he said. "I'm not doing anything other than playing." A Red with Efficiency, Mike described the enjoyment he gets from focusing on sailboat racing. "It's like nothing else matters," he said. "I can't do anything else the day of a race, and none of this tires me out. The focus gives me energy." This total engagement goes hand in hand with Reds' need for physical stimulation.

ENVIRONMENT AND PERSONAL CONNECTIONS

Reds take in the physical world around them—not in the quiet manner of Greens, who we'll meet in the next chapter, but in robust fashion. Where Greens merge, Reds surge. Reds have excellent observational and navigational skills that come with Extraverted Sensing, and they derive

Man consists of two parts, his mind and his body, only the body has more fun.

—Woody Allen

great enjoyment from them. They notice the small changes in a favorite trail hiked over and over—the changing color of the leaves, the stages of budding flowers. Reds see things in the physical world that elude the more Intuitive types.

As Mike described it: "I love seeing different things in the same place. I can hike up the same trail repeatedly for three weeks and it's always different—totally different!"

With few exceptions, Reds prefer physical activity with friends—it's a favorite way to connect with people. My brother Ronny has many friends, all of whom he met through sports. He ticked them off on his fingers: "Danny I met through football, Jim through basketball, Dick through basketball, Bob through racquetball. And Bill Russell—although we met when we were both playing for the Celtics, it was really through golf that we became friends." Several Reds have commented that what they miss when they are no longer playing on a team is the feeling of comraderie in the locker room before and after the game. As one Red former competitor said, "It was the twelve of us against the world."

Hugh said that with one exception, all of his friends are people he met through sports. I asked, given his knowledge of his own type, what advice he had for fellow ESFPs who want to bump up their activity. "I suggest they find other people at the same level," he said, "and activities that they can enjoy, together or as a group. If they're not at the same level, or if the level is too high, it's going to be discouraging and they're not going to do it."

Reds love games, sports, contests, and competitions—these are the ways they "play" in the world. They are restless indoors and need a playful environment, even at work. If they have gym equipment in the basement, chances are it doesn't see much action. Indoor exercise is far too routine and confining (unless it's being done as training for an outside event); it doesn't provide enough variety, challenge, or chances to use the skills Reds enjoy most.

Because Reds experience the world through their senses, not a sight or sound escapes their notice, and they're naturally aware of where they are in the physical world. Unlike some Intuitive types who can get lost in thought as well as in the woods, Reds easily navigate in unfamiliar environments and are not concerned about losing their way. They know they can get themselves back home, and they enjoy the adventure.

Being outdoors not only combats boredom, but Reds find the natural world to be a great stress reliever. Even cityscapes can do the trick. Natalie, a Red with Efficiency, is a retired realtor living in Manhattan. At the age of ninety-one, she still walks the city streets for two hours every day, regardless of the weather. She dresses appropriately, then heads out, pushing her walker with the built-in basket, feeling safe, unafraid of falling, and very much in the game. Many times during our interview, Natalie described how she dislikes being cooped up at home. "I get nervous sitting around," she said. "I get fidgety inside. I have to get out."

An indoor gym wouldn't do it for Natalie's Red personality. Walking the streets of New York City, energized by the sights, sounds, even the smells of the neighborhood, makes her feel alive and healthy. "I feel like I'm sixty," she said. "It makes all the difference."

If lifestyle requirements or training goals make indoor workouts necessary, Reds have better luck when they set themselves up near a bright open window with a great view. They can train with others, set up little competitions and short-term rewards, and blast their favorite music on their iPods to psych themselves up.

Even with their driving energy, Reds are easy-going and casual by nature. And they're among the most loyal of fans to their favorite sports teams. When Fall rolls around, it's easy to find them on weekends; if they're not out somewhere playing, they're in front of the TV set cheering their football team to victory.

Being with people who are responsive to this kind of enthusiasm—or who are equally as engaged in the activity—is energizing for this outgoing color. Reds enjoy playing hard with those who can join in with gusto. When training, they'll add a level of competition with teammates or friends to keep up the challenges and make the goals more real. They appreciate the support and the vitality that come from being active with companions, friends, and

---

Hours of boredom followed by sheer terror.

—Mike, Red with Efficiency, describing sailboat racing

teammates. Reds with Harmony look for a coach who is straightforward and encouraging. They want to know what he or she is going to do for them, including the skills they will learn.

Ronny played for the Celtics with team captain Bill Russell, under legendary coach Red Auerbach. I asked him what was great about the coach. He said Auerbach had been straightforward and clear. He told Ronny in bullet-like fashion, "Here's your role. One, Russell doesn't like anyone on his back. Two, be the first man back on defense, to keep people off Russell's back. Three, run like hell."

REDS WITH EFFICIENCY (ESTP)

Quick of step and speech, outgoing and persuasive, Reds with Efficiency do rather than ponder. With their shoot-from-the-hip approach, they are at their best when up against the wall. As Steve Myers described in *Influencing People Using Myers-Briggs* (p. 86), ESTPs are good at "solving urgent problems with proven methods." They analyze readily and keep the solution simple.

Reds with Efficiency are Introverted Thinkers; they analyze and consider the facts of a situation. They're not on the lookout for underlying meaning or complexity. In fact, hidden agendas don't occur to them. Common sense is highly valued, and they're proud of this quality in themselves. They want a clear, preferably short-term, goal, something they can readily shoot for and achieve.

This type is motivated by competition, which provides engagement, focus, and goals, spurring them on to train and achieve. "Winning, winning, winning—how many ways can I win?" said Mike of his enjoyment of competitive sailing. "You can be in the top ten; you can win in your class, your level; you can set a time and beat it. You can win your goals in so many ways. That's part of the fun."

Animated, charming, and excitable, Reds with Efficiency will do whatever it takes to maximize leisure time (and there's never enough!). When they're around, life is not dull.

Living life through their senses, Reds with Efficiency are drawn to activities involving speed and thrills and a challenge to their skills. To indulge this jump-in-with-both-feet personality, they actively seek out fast-paced experiences that make them feel alive. They're impatient with activities that move along slowly.

REDS WITH HARMONY (ESFP)

Like their Efficient color mates, Reds with Harmony are practical and realistic, living in the moment. They have keen senses through which they explore and experience the world. And there's so much to explore—Reds experience life as a sensory banquet.

But this is a much more people-focused type. Warm, generous, and fun-loving, Reds with Harmony want to share their irrepressible enthusiasm for life. They have no problem interacting with people of all ages, backgrounds, and cultures. They delight in being the center of attention, stimulating others to enjoy themselves, too. They have a gift for raising people's spirits and creating a fun-filled atmosphere.

Not surprisingly, with their love of the spotlight, they're lively conversationalists, quick with a joke or comeback. Reds with Harmony are typically uncomfortable with solitude for long periods and seek out the company of other people whenever they can find it. Gatherings are usually spontaneous, set up quickly and seamlessly. On any Saturday afternoon when the spirit hits, Karl makes a few calls to friends and in short order puts together a fun and fast-paced game of basketball at the local community center. His Red-with-Harmony preferences carry through to the rollicking gathering at his home afterward, complete with wings and pizza that seem to appear magically.

While Reds with Efficiency are motivated by a chance to win, Reds with Harmony focus on the fun. They love being physical with friends or other groups of people, as do Silvers with Harmony. "My idea of a perfect afternoon is to spend a few hours on Rollerblades with friends and then go out for a couple of margaritas," notes Karen.

Reds with Harmony naturally go with the flow and depend on their ability to improvise. They avoid structure and routine, and they're not known for long-range planning. Carefully groomed, they appreciate beauty and like to surround themselves with expansive views, open floor plans, good food, and good company.

As the famed character Auntie Mame announced to guests at one of her famous parties, "Live, live, live! Life is a banquet and most poor suckers are starving to death!"

MEET THE REDS

Tim, Red with Efficiency (ESTP)

Tim, at age thirty-one, is an investment consultant and a former professional triathlete. He now competes in state and regional triathlons and marathons and sees his current physical conditioning as supporting his life—professional, social, and family—rather than as the center of it.

In competition, Tim displays the all-or-nothing approach typical of Reds. He thrives on the exhilaration of being present and completely focused on the goals in front of him. Competition and the possibility of winning drive him to peak performance.

As Tim describes it: "If you're not competing, you're just going to accept ordinary effort. I always give one hundred percent. I always try my hardest." His competitive streak is intense: "I attack like I'm being chased. It's life or death. You must keep the attack on."

This "attack" suggests the kind of all-out energy Reds with Efficiency typically exert. There is an on/off aspect to their modus operandi that's exhilarating. It's what they look for in their physical outlets—especially in the "on" mode.

Red isn't just the color of fire, it's also the color of firefighters. Highly trained professionals, they spend endless hours at the firehouse, waiting, hanging out, talking, watching TV, reading, and maintaining their equipment. Then the alarm sounds—and physical inactivity becomes highest-level activity.

During his years in professional sports, Tim believed he had few limitations, and that hasn't changed. "I always wanted to be a world champion, to go to the Olympics, to be the best," he said. With a smile, he added, "I still don't rule myself out."

Randy, Red with Efficiency (ESTP)

Randy, a leadership and organizational consultant, is tall, muscular, and in top shape. He drives a red convertible, meticulously maintained, with over 120,000 miles on it. At nearly sixty years old (although you'd never guess his age), he mountain bikes and skis with much younger people. Randy began our interview by telling me that his wife (a Purple with Harmony) notices that he starts feeling poorly if he hasn't been outside and done something physically active. He went on to describe that being close to nature is of fundamental importance to him, and he can't get enough of it. He dresses for the outdoors and has to be in actual physical pain from the elements (e.g., frostbite) to stay indoors.

The only reason Randy works out indoors is so that he can do better outdoors. "I don't touch a Spinner bike in the summer when I can bike outside." He lifts weights only for the purpose of gaining strength so he can ski or bike better. He chooses Spinning classes carefully, avoiding those he considers "lollygagging." He needs to know the goal set for the class; for example, if there will be lots of climbing, hard flats, or intervals. Good music is mandatory; he likes rock and roll of the 60s and 70s.

Randy described the joy of breathing hard, getting his heart rate up to 75-to-90 percent of max, and listening to his own breath. When he's outside, his mind wanders, but he is very aware of where he is, noticing the quality of the road and the natural world around him.

Randy owns three bikes—a titanium road bike, a mountain bike, and an old one he rides on bike paths with the family. He is currently most enthusiastic about mountain biking and competes in several races and road hill climbs each season (including Mt. Washington). He enjoys the activity because he feels his technique is better than his strength, and technique is better suited for mountain biking, which involves getting over logs, around branches, and climbing. Road biking, in contrast, is a more constant, steady effort.

Reds with Efficiency are natural competitors and enjoy all the ways they can win or otherwise be successful. Randy laughed about all the little victories that are so enjoyable to him. He was careful to note that competition is fun and provides a goal, but he hates ugly competition or winning at all costs. "Up a hill, there's this guy I want to take out, or I pick out a hill climb and say to someone, 'You're not going to let me get by you.' I try my hardest to drop somebody. At sixty, it's fun to be better than guys much younger than me."

Randy told me that on Sunday he would be biking with a group. I was curious why he'd go with others and how he approached a group outing. "It happens very easily—on Tuesday, I put an e-mail out to friends with the idea: 'Anyone up for a little day trip to the Kingdom Trails on Sunday? Forecast: Sunny!' I like to leave it open and flexible so people can change their mind if a better option comes up."

He said it's fun to mountain bike with a group because it's "more stop and go," which makes for lots of what he described as sensory conversations. Examples include: "What do you think about that section of the trail?" "Were you able to get over that rock pile without putting a foot down [stopping]?" and "How is your new bike performing?"

Randy enjoys maintaining his bikes in perfect condition. During the summer, the cars are outside the garage and the bikes are in so he can work on them. He commented that biking provides him two things he loves, "Breathing hard and taking apart something and putting it back together."

At the end of our interview, I asked him about biking and fun. "If it wasn't fun, I wouldn't do it. I come home, I have blood on my elbows, my knees are skinned, my bike's a mess, and I look like hell. My wife says, 'You call that fun?'" With a big smile, he answered, "Yes!"

Karen, Red with Harmony (ESFP)

One of my earliest interview subjects, Karen is a veterinarian who maintains a busy practice in her rural community. My first question to her was, "What motivates you to exercise?"

"The thought never crossed my mind," she said. "Sports is just what I do with other people. If I run, I feel better. Breathing hard is positive. Staying in shape has always been important—it's not about being fast."

Sports were less about competing than about having fun with her wide circle of friends, but the thought of besting someone was not out of the question. She relishes her skills and enjoys an opportunity to strut her stuff, even if she is the only one who knows it. She described an example using the colorful language characteristic of Reds: "A little light goes off when I'm skiing down a mountain past a young guy, knowing that I'm dusting his butt."

Karen said there's no such thing as a typical week of exercise. She'll respond to a last-minute invitation with little hesitation.

"There's no such thing as 'typical,' but I can talk about yesterday," she said. "When I woke up, I thought I might spend some time gardening. But a friend called asking me to go sailing. So, with two kayaks on the roof of the car and our bikes and dogs in tow, my friend and I headed for Lake Champlain. I took along the kayaks in case we were too late to go out sailing. No sense getting all upset and blowing the whole opportunity."

She described the back seat of her car where she keeps her Rollerblades, a wet suit, a dry suit, and a wind shirt. "I keep it all there so I can just walk out of the house and be ready," she said.

Karen's many activities include horseback riding, skiing (with the ski patrol), and skating. She described the ski area on Friday night as an "extended family," echoing the sentiments of Susanne, a Silver with Harmony, regarding her running friends. These are the two types that most often report enjoying activities with groups; the camaraderie of games and sports appeals to these playful types.

Karen is ready for anything. She maintains an active lifestyle by being responsive to the moment. And as she will tell you, anything can happen in the moment.

John, Red with Harmony (ESFP)

"If it's not play, if it's not fun, I won't do it."

John's approach to fitness has Red with Harmony written all over it. He doesn't think in terms of exercise, but rather talks about play and sports and engaging in activities. "It's boring to just stay in shape," he said. "I need to have a great end goal."

When asked about a typical week of activity, he piped right up: "My sport is snowboarding," he said. All his physical activity, including off-season pursuits, is aimed at remaining in shape for snowboarding. "In the summer, I keep myself tuned up for winter," he said.

Although John isn't interested in exercise for its own sake, he'll do what it takes in the service of something else—in this case, getting out on the slopes and riding. With his dedication to a high-energy, quick-response sport like snowboarding, the motivation to stay in shape year round is strong, and John fills his summers with biking, in-line skating, and pickup games of racquetball so he doesn't lose his edge.

John rides his snowboard for six or seven months out of the year in the northern New England region where he lives. "I go out every weekend from October to April," he said. "One year, I was able to snowboard until May."

John didn't choose snowboarding; snowboarding chose him. He was once an Alpine skier, but needed new equipment one year and said he was beginning to tire of the downhill sport. "I was losing interest, so I tried something new, and I liked it," he said.

When he's out on the snow, John enjoys being with others who are also experiencing the thrill and skill of snowboarding down a steep mountainside. "I like other people in the environment," he said. "It's not something I do with friends, but when I'm out there, if other people are there, it's great."

If he went boarding with a group, he said he'd feel obliged to stay with them, which would be too confining. He prefers being free to go off on new trails and explore unknown terrain from time to time. Chatting casually with other skiers and boarders on the lifts and slopes provides enough contact to satisfy him. John likes the easy camaraderie and enjoys giving people tips on their technique, but he doesn't have to "hang" with anyone during his rides. "I don't rely on anybody else," he said.

Maintaining the freedom to explore and experience new sensations is important to John, who stays in the moment when he's out playing in nature. He doesn't bother with a gym or fitness center. During the summer, one of his favorite activities is skating on a bike path. "I notice the people, the lake, the whole environment," he said. "And I pay close attention to the condition of the path because it affects my balance. I am definitely not spacing out or in a zone."

Asked about whether he puts limits on himself when he's in the middle of an extreme sport, John answered that he's careful about risky behavior. While other types might perceive his activities as dangerous, John disagrees. "I'm on the cautious side," he said. "I know my limits, my boundaries. I don't go beyond my skill level."

John said he can't sit still for long. At home, he gets antsy with inactivity and has to get up, wash the car, take the dog for a walk, or get out to do…something!

FAVORITE ACTIVITIES

Basketball: Fast-paced, this sport appeals to Red's enjoyment of focus and split-second timing. Casually planned or impromptu pick-up games are a good way to spend time with friends.

Biking: Mountain or road biking is a beautiful way for Reds to be outside, enjoy the view, get their heart-rate up, spend time with friends, and explore new areas. It involves minimal process and can be a great way to commute.

Hiking and climbing: Reds are never bored outside. Hiking and climbing provide great opportunities to get outdoors and notice all variations in the landscape.

In-line skating: The strength and balance required by Rollerblades are challenges to Reds, while the fast pace gets the heart rate up. And the fluid movement is enjoyable.

Racquetball: Fast-paced, intense, and high energy, this game appeals to stimulus-hungry Reds.

Skiing or snowboarding: The balance and finesse needed for both sports are natural skills for Reds. They enjoy the flow and rhythms of the ride and the views. The playful aspect of snowboarding holds particular appeal.

Tennis: Energetic and calling for quick reflexes, this game lets Reds play at many levels. Courts are readily available at playgrounds, parks, and schoolyards.

ROADBLOCKS AND TIPS

Roadblocks

- Finding "exercise" tedious
- Not having goals in sight
- Inaccessibility to outdoors
- Lack of people to "play" with

Top 10 Tips

1. You are likely to be bored with pure exercise. Stay in shape by choosing activities and sports that are fun and can be done with others.

2. Train for an event with others. The event provides motivation and energy for peak performance, and fellow trainers make it fun.

3. Maintain a network of active people who you can contact and who will contact you for physical activity and sports together.

4. Create mini-goals along the way, such as time, distance, or improvement. Provide tangible rewards for yourself and others. A promised get-together after a game, for example, is a treat after a strenuous workout.

5. Get outside. With your outstanding observation and navigation skills, you won't be bored in outdoor settings, which will provide the stimulation to keep you going.

6. Keep momentum up by having your goals in sight. Post notes, action pictures, and other reminders of what you want to achieve. Keep gear handy so you will be ready for action when an opportunity opens up.

7. If you use indoor equipment, find or move it near a window so you can enjoy views of nature and outdoor activity.

8. Keep your iPod handy and filled with your favorite music to keep you going, especially when exercising inside.

9. To avoid injury, resist your natural impulse to "go all out" every time. Go easy when rehabbing from an injury or getting back in shape.

10. Avoid making commitments that impinge on your inclination toward freedom and flexibility. You are unlikely to sustain workouts over-scheduled with others.

RED WORDS

Action, all-out, fast, flexible, fun, goals, hands-on, nimble, observant, play, restless, speed, stimulation, thrills, variety

Reds at a Glance—Roaring Reds: Now!

ESTP: Red Efficiency—Dominant Extraverted Sensing with Auxiliary Introverted Thinking

ESFP: Red Harmony—Dominant Extraverted Sensing with Auxiliary Introverted Feeling

Overall Qualities	Like a siren in a chase, Reds love to be where the action is. Reds experience life through their senses, craving stimulation and adventure from the physical world. Moving is natural; physical activity is about being alive. While Reds are oriented to activity in the physical world, the idea of putting time aside for "exercise" seems tedious and boring. Reds understand the importance of fitness and incorporate it in their playful and physically active lifestyle.
Motivation:	• Enjoyment of highly stimulating activities • Finding physical activity to be fun • Inspired by performance • Competition with a shot at winning
Approach:	• Playful • Enjoy mini-competitions—with many ways to win • Give it their all, every time • Casual, spontaneous, go with the flow • Enjoy variety of activities • Keep equipment/gear handy

Focus:	• Attention is in the moment • Quick responders • Enjoy using their outstanding navigational and observational skills • Goal provides focus—boring to just stay in shape • IPod loaded with energetic music or television turned on when engaged in repetitious cardio activities
Environments:	• High energy and action-packed setting • Outdoors provides stimulation • Enjoy observing small details in nature • Gym—equipment with a view
Interpersonal Connections:	• Train for a goal/event with others • Energy diminishes when alone • Enjoy games/activities/sports with others • Inspired to better performance by competitions
Sample Quotes:	*Routine exercise is boring and I'm unsuccessful at it. Competing is at the center of my motivation. If I'm not competing, I'm just going to accept ordinary effort. I approach every race with the feeling I have a chance to win. If I don't think I have a chance to win, it's no fun. I have to have a goal.* Red Efficiency *Yesterday I planned to work in the garden, but a friend called— "Let's go kayaking!" So off we went to the lake with our kayaks and our dogs. For me, there's no such thing as an exercise routine. I keep Rollerblades, a wet suit, and dry clothing in the car so I'm always ready for action.* Red Harmony

CHAPTER 6

ISP, Greener than Green: Nature Beckons

ISTP: Dominant Introverted Thinking with Auxiliary Extraverted Sensing
ISFP: Dominant Introverted Feeling with Auxiliary Extraverted Sensing

What color but Green, the color of nature, could represent these lovers of all outdoors? If Greens could live in full accordance with their true selves, they would have little need for planned exercise. Getting outside is their priority, and physical activity is both an excuse for and a benefit of doing so. Being outside lets Greens know they're alive, so ready access to the outdoors is a basic necessity.

Greens are highly attuned to and observant of the physical world around them. Their profound attention to detail and their observational skills influence all aspects of what they do and when they do it. A great example is night driving: Many people avoid it for various reasons—they're distracted by oncoming lights, their vision is limited, they don't like to drive when they're fatigued. But as one Green said, "Night driving in Vermont is simply a waste of time. When it's dark, you can't see the landscape."

Their demeanor is understated, quiet, and unobtrusive. In groups, Greens tend toward the background, preferring others to take the lead in social interactions. This is especially true in situations that are more about small talk, where the objectives are not clear.

Their close identification with the physical world is reflected in their wardrobes. They dress comfortably and simply, preferring soft tones, natural textiles, and comfortable shoes. Greens choose clothes that help them blend in and merge with the physical world.

As parents, they describe their most pleasurable times with their children as those spent sharing their deep enjoyment of the physical world and encouraging their children to appreciate it as they do. As Dave, a Green with Efficiency, notes, "Pure recreation is going out with the kids and picking up rocks, bugs, and salamanders."

Never bored outside and frequently bored inside, Greens do all they can to bring the outdoors in. They add large picture windows and decks to their homes, and they seek natural construction materials such as wood and stone. A Green's work environment includes pictures of waterfalls, sunsets, sunrises, and canyons. Andrew Wyeth was often mentioned as a favorite landscape artist, but don't expect to see his prints displayed in fancy frames.

Greens might also have rock collections or driftwood sculptures—anything real or realistic.

MOTIVATION, APPROACH, FOCUS

With the reserved demeanor of Introverts, Greens are quiet observers of the physical world. Nature *is* their nature. Many report getting antsy, irritable, and depressed when they don't get enough outside time. Considering that they're also very practical, it makes sense to get their exercise within the activities of daily living, outdoors as much as possible.

Regimented indoor exercise according to a fixed schedule falls somewhere along a continuum between *turn-off* and *torture*. Their natural physicality inclines Greens to main-

tain a baseline of physical fitness, but incorporating a regimented training program into their lives is unlikely to happen without a specific reason—such as getting in shape to fully enjoy a favorite outdoor activity, or to achieve a prized goal, like being part of a climbing or backpacking expedition.

Greens avoid indoor gyms, only using them to increase their stamina for an important outdoor challenge. Chris, a Green with Harmony, said he prefers running in a park to the city streets. And unless the weather is really hostile, he hikes and bikes during the summer and snowshoes and cross-country skis in winter. "Going to a gym to work out was really difficult for me, so I stopped going, and now I do one hundred percent of my physical activity outdoors," he said.

Greens' personality is casual, and they enjoy opportunities that let them spontaneously respond and adapt to environmental callings and challenges. They're quick-thinking in crisis situations. They value being prepared, anticipating and analyzing risks and, most importantly, being effectively self-reliant.

When Greens match their lifestyle to their personality, they have no problem getting all the exercise they need. Paul, a Green with Efficiency, worked in his yard sawing branches, pruning trees, and tending his garden. For the fifty years he practiced law in a downtown firm, he walked a mile to work most days, even walking home for lunch.

John, a Green with Harmony, is an outdoor educator in his state. He volunteers with his local division of the Appalachian Trail Club. For more than thirty years, he's been part of a team that maintains the woodland trails, digging ditches, clearing debris, and removing rocks from the trails. Free weights and treadmills just can't compete.

ENVIRONMENT AND PERSONAL CONNECTIONS

With calm acceptance, Greens embrace the outdoors in all its conditions. They don't complain or moan about the weather being uncooperative, but merely adapt to it. With boots and another layer of clothing, they are undaunted by rain or a drop in temperature that would cause other types to change their plans. Greens are not mall walkers.

Too much time inside is stressful for Greens. Getting outside gives them an opportunity to clear their minds and wrestle with the energizing and calming challenges of nature. Almost any outdoor environment will do—woods, mountains, lakes, oceans, beaches, trails, river walks, and parks. However, Greens have a special affinity for water. Many talk about their love of surfing, windsurfing, swimming, snorkeling, and scuba diving. Yet I have not come across a single Green who swims in an indoor, chlorinated pool. What could be more unnatural?

They're so highly attuned to taking in every natural detail around them that many Greens, like Reds, say they enjoy hiking their favorite trails frequently. They find something new and different every time.

With such keen observation and orienting skills, Greens have an exceptional capacity for navigating in unfamiliar terrain, showing little concern about going off the beaten path. "Do you ever get lost in the woods?" I asked Garn, a Green-with-Harmony college student. "No, I always know where I am," he said. "Images of the trail are in my brain, I carry a compass, and I have contour maps burned into memory. I never get lost."

I like all exercise outdoors, even in a torrential downpour. Indoors does nothing for me.

—Leonard, Green with Harmony

Nicole, a career Coastguard officer, Green with Harmony, had a similar response: "Places are like a grid in my brain," she said. "I have an innate ability to find my way around. I enjoy getting lost and trying to find my way back." After hearing such tales from Green after Green, I started referring to this color as the GPS of personality types.

During the course of my research, many members of this color type spoke affectionately of the outdoor decks attached to their homes. Observing the pattern, I wondered how this might be an expression of type. I asked Chris, a Green with Harmony, "What is it about decks that you find so appealing?"

"It's the sensory intake," he said. "Decks give you the view, and you've got to get the view."

For a meeting with Jim, a Green with Harmony who owns a woodworking shop where he handcrafts rocking chairs, we sat out on his expansive deck to talk. Walking through Jim's house on the way to the deck, I looked around at the furnishings—lots of wood, with natural stone in every room. Large windows looked out on views of the mountains in all directions. At the end of our interview, I asked him about his deck.

"I love it," he said, and showed me plans to double the size of the already large deck we sat on. In fact, construction was underway.

Of all the color types, Greens report the most significant preference for solo physical activity. Time alone with nature recharges their batteries. Alone, Greens can directly connect with nature and enjoy the quiet sounds, smells, and views with no need to converse, coordinate, or adapt to someone else.

Jim, the Green with Harmony woodworker, described his hikes: "I don't like to walk and talk," he said. "So I mostly hike by

I do four miles every day. It takes me an hour and fifteen minutes. I have two routes, alternating them and reversing direction, which gives me a total of four different walks. I always take binoculars, and I identify plants, birds, and animals along the way. When reversed, these are completely different walks, and I see completely different things.

—Ellie, Green with Harmony

myself. Sometimes I go with my brother, but we understand each other. We usually hike about twenty feet apart. We know we're not going to talk."

This preference for solo activity stems from many aspects of Greens' personality. For one, going it alone minimizes the need for coordination and advance planning with other people. Being alone lets them catch the moment as it arises, without checking with anyone else. It speaks to the casual and flexible world that Greens prefer—minimalist and responsive to the conditions of the moment.

Alone, too, Greens can directly connect with their surroundings. As one Green said, "When I'm riding a bike, there's so much to see and experience. The farm smells and the tree smells. It's so meaningful."

Alexis, a Green with Efficiency, describes going out alone in the fresh snow. "It's quiet, the trees are still, nothing is moving—it's just the snow," she said. Hiking in the woods, she enjoys looking for animals, noticing the rocks, where the trees have fallen, how wide the path is compared to other trails. "I love taking it all in," she said.

Greens enjoy the idea of being in good physical shape—maintaining a baseline level of fitness—so they can participate in the activities they find most meaningful. When training is needed for a specific event, they'll design their own schedules and work on them independently out of an inner desire to meet their goals. Training with others doesn't motivate them, and exercise buddies hold little appeal.

GREENS WITH EFFICIENCY

Greens with Efficiency are men and women of few words. When they speak, they're brief and to the point. Why say something in two hundred words that can be said in twenty? They're not sidetracked by what-ifs, but like to move forward in a linear fashion. They're minimalist and resourceful and are natural troubleshooters.

> *When I'm hiking, it's gratifying to see the deer and turkeys and other wild birds, but it's much more fun to get to the top of the mountain. That's when you really see something. Looking out at the horizon you can see over everything. It's that perspective—it's just beautiful.*
>
> *—Ann, Green with Harmony*

You can count on a Green with Efficiency to look for the most direct route to all things—including exercise. Why set aside extra time for exercise when you can include it in household duties, yard chores, and all the many activities of daily living? It's practical, and Greens with Efficiency are nothing if not practical. Their sensible and efficient natures are offended by the thought of driving to a gym and paying to use a treadmill when they can walk up and down hills. They won't hire someone to clear the debris or dig the ditch in front of their house when they can do it themselves and get an upper body and leg workout at the same time.

Greens with Efficiency enjoy challenging themselves with intensity and competition. Ellen described her college days playing field hockey as "fun, and I enjoyed being held accountable." She thrived on being held to a high standard, and she contrasted field hockey with her enjoyment of hiking. "Hiking is on my own—no need to be held accountable."

Greens with Efficiency often report this level of response to intensity and challenge. Dave describes his own rigorous training for the dangerous and demanding climb to the top of Alaska's Mt. Denali as exhilarating.

Part of what he enjoyed about the experience was learning to use the specialized equipment necessary to make the climb.

Like their Red with Efficiency counterparts, Greens with Efficiency are Introverted Thinkers. This predisposes them to puzzle out and solve practical and mechanical problems. Perhaps that's why they are known for their love of tools; they appreciate how much they can accomplish with something as simple as a hand saw. They can fix almost anything, or at least accurately diagnose the problem. They seek freedom to use their analytical skills to figure things out, and they're at their best when they are left on their own to do so. They're patient with a problem to solve. You won't find Greens with Efficiency tempted to throw a troublesome computer against the wall. The machine is doing what machines do, and there is no reason to get riled up.

Greens' natural readiness is appreciated by their office mates. They're the go-to people for help with computer problems, jammed windows, broken furniture, or tire changes. You can count on them to keep a stash of simple tools in their desk—including duct tape—ready to come to the rescue with the simplest solution.

GREENS WITH HARMONY

While Greens with Efficiency use their analytical skills to make decisions, Greens with Harmony are guided by their inner values. A gentle love of nature and a reverence for "all creatures great and small" are hallmarks of their personality. They have an easygoing appreciation for the outdoors that doesn't require the engagement aimed at accomplishing a goal that so frequently attracts Greens with Efficiency.

A calm exterior and affinity for physical environments are at the core of their personality. Greens with Harmony have simple needs, and their minimalist nature inclines them to live with less. What they do appreciate is a house built with stone and wood, and a deck with natural vistas. And they'll save up for a river-rafting trip to Montana with a few good friends.

Greens with Harmony are Introverted Feelers, inclining them to be caring and practical. They have a knack for providing the perfect hands-on help at just the right moment—whether it be cleaning the trout in time for pan frying or quietly gathering sticks at the beach to roast marshmallows. They have an uncanny ability to assess the needs of a situation and take care of the simple tasks that are easily overlooked by others.

With this inclination to care for others, Greens with Harmony say time alone in nature allows them to soak up the beauty around them without the temptation to respond to someone else's needs. They can come back from a hike or bike alone recharged and unburdened.

Greens with Harmony have a friendly laugh, and people find them accessible. Interactions tend to be congenial—but brief. That is, unless they're talking about something real and physical that they love. They can wax long on the subject of snow blanketing the frozen beaver ponds after a storm in winter, for example.

Greens with Harmony tend to avoid competitive sports, and many describe unpleasant experiences in high school as part of a team. Their love of nature gets them out of the house and on the trails, paths, and waterways with no urging.

MEET THE GREENS

Steve, Green with Efficiency (ISTP)

Steve is a classic man of few words, but when he speaks, people perk up and listen. In conversation, as in life, he is practical and direct. Tall and lanky, Steve maintains a high level of fitness, but it's unnatural for him to set time aside for exercise. Instead, he builds it into the rest of his life.

"I like the idea of being fit, but I don't make time for it, except in connection with something practical," he said. "For instance, I park a mile from work and walk the rest of the way. It saves money and I get my exercise." This is a lifestyle practice he has maintained for twenty years working in a downtown office.

Steve's first career was in diesel mechanics, but he later went on to become a CPA. He now owns an accounting business that specializes in commercial real estate services. Steve is married and the father of six children.

Exercise comes into the picture for Steve as a component of other activities he's involved in. "I enjoy exercise if I'm doing physical work that is production oriented," he said. "I work around the yard, saw branches, prune, work in the garden. These things I relish." The typical activities of a busy day help him with basic physical maintenance, and late at night he enjoys a quiet walk under the stars—probably his time to ponder.

Only when he has a particular physical aim—increasing stamina and strength for hiking and hunting, for instance—will Steve consider scheduling training time.

"I want to be strong for deer camp," Steve said. "I've never been successful with indoor, repetitious exercise, but I'll think about it if it will help me hike better and improve my endurance during hunting season. That interests me."

Preferring to be outdoors as much as possible, Steve hunts in the fall, walks year round, and hikes and snowshoes in the woods near his house, finding ways to get outside in all seasons. "I enjoy extended time in the woods," he said.

Dave, Green with Efficiency (ISTP)

Dave is a forty-year-old college administrator. A few years ago, he fulfilled a major life ambition and took part in an expedition to climb the highest peak in North America, Alaska's Mt. Denali.

What was behind this Green with Efficiency's adventure of epic proportions, I wondered. Dave easily ticked off his motivations: "It was the adventure, the cold, the challenge, the danger, and the extreme of things." He went on: "I find risk factors exhilarating. I like to analyze risks, understand the dangers involved, and prepare for them. I like being on the edge, but controlling the edge. Having to be rescued is a failure."

As a Green with Efficiency, Dave typically is not inclined toward routine exercise on an ongoing basis, but there's nothing typical or routine about training for such an adventure. With a goal of that magnitude to prepare for, Dave described enjoying the training process.

"I liked the preparation process for Mt. Denali; the training was physical and technical—all the stuff, the gear, preparing for the climatic changes. It was very interesting." As part of his training, Dave exercised on a StairMaster several days a week, regularly increasing the incline as he added weight to his backpack, until he was able to carry fifty-five pounds for an extended period of time.

Reflecting on the Denali climb, Dave described long periods of boredom mixed in with some very scary moments. Among the enduring rewards of the expedition is the knowledge that he was able do it. One climber's online journal mentioned that there are more than three hundred tourists and guides on Mt. Denali at one time, and only a handful of them make it to the top. Dave said he was satisfied that he wasn't the best, but he was among the best—in his words, "in the top 20 percent," those who went all the way. The biggest reward for him was reaching the top of the highest peak in North America to see panoramic views of Alaska's wild and frozen terrain stretching out below.

Dave's Denali climb was a "once in a lifetime experience." On a more regular basis, his lifestyle is anything but sedentary and includes bike riding to and from work, Telemark skiing, hiking, other rugged outdoor activities, and fun challenges.

As a busy dad, Dave tries to juggle his much-needed time alone with the responsibilities of work and family. On one weekend morning, he squeezed in a brisk jog up a nearby mountain, 4,400 feet to the summit. To increase the challenge, he zipped his arms inside his jacket and "ran armless." He was proud that he made it to the top in one hour and fifteen minutes. "There were eight inches of snow on the ground," he said. "It was so beautiful. I just sat there."

Dave enjoys spending active time outdoors with his children. He is pleased to be able to pass on his skills and love of nature. "With my kids, preparing them for survival in the wilderness is fun!" he said.

"I'm always outside doing stuff," he said. "If I don't get outside, I become moody and antsy. My work deteriorates and I can't concentrate. My body has to be at a certain level so I can do what I want to do."

Todd, Green with Harmony (ISFP)

Todd is a Hollywood actor and stuntman. He's on movie sets most days of the week and describes his work as "physically demanding and fun"—perfect for a Green. Todd keeps himself in peak condition to handle the many feats and stunts required in his work—fighting with other men, falling into airbags and boxes, crashing cars, and crashing bikes. He talked about his work with energy and enthusiasm. "Cars are fun, car chases are fun, fights are fun…like a dance."

Todd stays in shape not by working out at the gym but through the activities he loves. "I am completely turned off when someone suggests that we meet at the gym at seven a.m. to lift weights," he said. "That kind of exercise seems never-ending, and I hate never-ending things. I need to know there's a goal, otherwise it feels joyless."

Todd spoke warmly as he described his enjoyment of the outdoors.

"I love hiking by myself," he said. "I love being in nature. Hiking clears my head. I can do the same hike fifty times and see different animals, different flora…something different around the bend." He occasionally hikes the hills with his wife and a few other people, urging them to reach the peak. As a Green, getting to the top and enjoying the view is the reward. Others don't always see it that way. "I go to the top 100 percent of the time," Todd said. "My wife turns around a few minutes from the top. I don't get it. It's baffling."

In addition to hiking and rock climbing—another favorite of Todd's—he enjoys surfing in the ocean not far from his home. He is out on the water every chance he gets. "Every wave is different, and I paddle out as far as I can," he said. "I particularly love it when no one is around."

Todd grew up in Vermont, and, having a father who was a ski coach, he's a skilled skier. He takes advantage of every opportunity to hit the mountain trails by himself. Aware of his tendency to want to please others around him—a notable Green with Harmony characteristic—skiing alone removes that temptation.

A typical Green, Todd is naturally active and described having difficultly sitting around doing nothing. He prefers living outdoors as much as possible. Our interview was conducted over the phone. I had already interviewed a number of Greens with Harmony and I had become curious about their commonly expressed love of outdoor decks. At the end of the interview, I asked Todd if his home happened to have a deck. With a hearty laugh, he answered, "Do you think I would be talking to you for an hour if I wasn't sitting on my deck? If I were inside, I would be very anxious to have this interview over!"

Katie, Green with Harmony (ISFP)

Katie lives in a townhouse in Bucks County, Pennsylvania, where she has easy access to the outdoors and hiking trails in her rural area. Typical of her Green-with-Harmony personality, being outside is what drives her. "Exercise is a vehicle for getting me into nature," Katie said. "I don't go outside to get exercise—the exercise is secondary. The only way I like to exercise is if I'm doing it for a purpose—and if it's outside."

Immediately upon moving into her townhouse, she replaced all the windows with new ones twice as big. Her walls are covered with posters and prints of the Grand Canyon and the wide open spaces of Arizona. Many of her nature prints feature waterscapes, and she's especially fond of Maxfield Parish prints of water and rock. Her office also has walls decorated with natural prints. Throughout the townhouse, Katie has six water fountains, some of which she built herself. There's a working fountain in every room.

Katie commutes to her job as a social worker in Trenton, New Jersey, four days a week, leaving her free to kayak the other three days. Traveling to the water is part of the fun, she said, and kayaking has enabled her to see much of the country. "It's a view you can't get from hiking—it's another perspective."

During summers, Katie can kayak closer to home on the Delaware River—a Class II waterway. There she can hone her skills, going out without paddles, practicing her rolls to be ready for more challenging trips. "I don't get scared if I'm ready to handle risks," she said.

Going out on white water is less about strength than about timing, agility, and stability, says Katie. "It's not a muscle sport, but a *finesse* sport. When you're kayaking, you are part of the water—you become the water."

Katie has always been deeply immersed in activities she loves. As a young girl growing up in rural Pennsylvania, she loved horses. "I was one of those horse crazy kids," she said. "My parents bought me a horse, and I showed horses until I was fourteen. I loved being around the stable. I loved the horsey smell."

When the family moved to Alabama, she no longer had a horse of her own, but she remained involved. "I took a year off from school between high school and college that became six years," she said. "I became an exercise rider for Thoroughbreds. I loved being outside with the horses. I loved trail riding and fox hunting [she was careful to explain that no foxes were killed] in the beauty of open country."

As a Green with Harmony, Katie has a preference for keeping plans open-ended and unstructured. The kayaking group she travels with fits into this model.

"That's what I love about the group," she said. "You don't make plans. You don't know the river levels ahead of time. You might not even know where you're heading. You have to see what's running, then make decisions. I'm not one of the deciders, and I like that. Some people are deciders—some aren't. But suddenly, there's a plan."

Katie takes pains to keep herself healthy and in shape with proper diet and by watching her weight. She tries to eat an organic and chemical-free diet, and she uses biodegradable materials as much as she can in her life. Under her bed, she stows a Nordic Track, which she uses occasionally while watching television. It's the television show she's focused on—that engages her mind—during the time she exercises on the track. In her kitchen, she keeps a small trampoline near a window looking out onto the sun porch. She jumps on that, usually while she's doing something else, like preparing a meal.

Katie said her mood actually suffers if she doesn't get out enough. "I get antsy, edgy, and irritable," she said. "It's not just doing something outside—it's being outside, even sitting by a creek with the dog." She considers outdoor activity an integral aspect of her life, and she could not imagine someone of her type who didn't.

FAVORITE ACTIVITIES

Activities of daily living: Greens appreciate parking farther from a destination and walking instead of driving; taking the stairs instead of the elevator; maintaining the yard: cleaning up brush, chopping wood, putting up fences, or spreading compost on the vegetable garden. Taking care of the home environment is not only convenient, but also provides many opportunities to be active and maintain fitness.

Biking: Solo rides provide the best opportunity to savor the experience, whether road biking or mountain biking. Practical Greens can ride a bike to work instead of driving.

Hiking/climbing: Alone or with one or two quiet friends, packing only what they need, Greens keep hiking simple. Hike the back country, or reach the top of a mountain where the view is the payoff. Keep it convenient by scouting out local trail systems; many towns and cities maintain them in public parks.

Horseback riding: While riding provides exercise, all aspects of the horsey life are appealing—grooming the horse, mucking the stables, carrying water and feed, pitching hay—especially to Greens with Harmony.

Running: Greens love the opportunity to get outside, run through changing vistas, down the path into the park, away from traffic. Running is also convenient and can be done alone.

Skiing/snowshoeing: Snow trails in back country take Greens into the winter woods, away from people and city sounds. Alpine skiing provides magnificent views, with new vistas appearing at every turn. Weekday outings mean fewer crowds.

Swimming and scuba diving: Greens have a special attraction to water—rivers, waterfalls, gorges, ponds, and streams. Divers find an entire underwater world to explore in oceans and deepwater lakes. But their sensitivity to unnatural chlorinated pools makes swimming indoors unappealing.

Walking: Any bit of nature will do. Most cities now set aside natural reserves where people can enjoy flora and fauna away from the sights ands sounds of traffic and congestion. With outstanding observational skills, Greens enjoy detecting the small and spectacular physical changes that are always there to be found. Binoculars can make it more fun.

Windsurfing/sailboarding: These activities bring Greens as close to nature as they can get, merging with the water and the wind. Challenging and thrilling, they combine all the elements that appeal to Greens—sensory experience, alone time, and the natural world.

ROADBLOCKS AND TIPS

Roadblocks:

- Inaccessibility of nature
- Failure to have a routine that can include activities of daily life
- Finding "exercise" tedious
- Difficulty finding time alone

Top 10 Tips

1. Investigate nature preserves, bike paths, and river walks near work and home. Don't be discouraged if the back yard doesn't open onto a nature reserve; the great outdoors might be closer than you think.

2. Find natural and convenient ways to include exercise in the activities of daily living rather than as add-ons—yard work, housework, walking to destinations, and using stairs instead of elevators are all good. You'll appreciate the practicality and simplicity of achieving two aims with one activity.

3. Create time alone for the important balance and productivity it brings to your life. Negotiate work and family responsibilities to ensure that time.

4. Enjoy nature in all its forms and at all times of day. Rise early to enjoy the sunrise. Go out for a walk, run, swim, or bike ride. Don't rule out nighttime; it provides one more opportunity with another set of sensations.

5. With your love of vistas and views, make sure you go to the top. That's what makes it worth the climb.

6. Participate in hands-on volunteer activities as a way to give back to the community while gaining physical benefits from the exercise involved. Offering to help maintain the grounds at a playground or park or working on the nature trails are other ways to enjoy physical activity while being productive.

7. Share your love of the outdoors with children. Lead your child's scouting troop, coach their teams, and get outside with them. Teaching a mountaineering or nature course might also be right up your alley.

8. Train for an outdoor challenge or meaningful activity by yourself. You're not the "exercise buddy" type. Create your own training plan and enjoy yourself.

9. Revisit favorite places. Enjoy noticing physical changes, both big and small.

10. Bring the binoculars, camera, or compass—these items make your time outside even more fun and fascinating.

GREEN WORDS

Alone, analytical, calm, casual, friendly, goals, minimalist, nature, observant, outdoors, practical, preparation, quiet, resourceful, vistas, water

Greens at a Glance—Greener than Green: Nature Beckons

ISTP: Green Efficiency—Dominant Introverted Thinking with Auxiliary Extraverted Sensing

ISFP: Green Harmony—Dominant Introverted Feeling with Auxiliary Extraverted Sensing

Overall Qualities	The natural world beckons. Greens seamlessly merge with the physical world. Being outside makes them feel alive. Greens are naturally observant of the concrete details and small variations in their environment. With their minimalist nature and practical approach, getting their exercise through activities of daily living, including working outside, makes sense. Greens are motivated to maintain a level of fitness so they can participate in the outdoor activities and challenges that are important to them.
Motivation:	• Getting outside, more important than the activity • Being outside to recharge their batteries—too much inside time is stressful • Increasing stamina to fully enjoy meaningful outdoor activities • Increasing ability to risks effectively, to be prepared and self-reliant
Approach:	• Establish easy access to nature, able to easily respond to "need" to get outdoors • Spontaneously respond to environmental callings • Include exercise as part of physically active lifestyle—practical • Minimalist in all things

Focus:	• Attention to what's in front of them in the moment • Naturally take in the physical surroundings, including smells and sounds • Details and small variations in nature
Environments:	• Enjoy using outstanding navigational skills—the GPSs of the type world • Accept nature on its own terms and embrace all weather conditions and all outdoors—sun, rain, snow, woods, mountain, lakes, and ocean. • Views and vistas • Will train at fitness center in preparation for an outdoor event that is important to them
Interpersonal Connections:	• Significant preference for being alone and experiencing the physical world without the distraction of conversation • Solo experiences allow flexibility • Prefer to train for a goal alone • Participate quietly alongside others
Sample Quotes:	*I like the idea of being fit, but I don't make time unless it's in connection with a practical activity. For instance, I park a mile from work. I save money and get exercise along the way. Repetitive exercise in a gym is hard to confront. I enjoy the woods. I'm never bored outdoors.* *Green Efficiency* *I love being in nature … surfing in the ocean, rock climbing, skiing, and hiking. When biking, I always take binoculars and identify plants, birds, and animals along the way. I prefer to be by myself. I have the tendency to please and that's not there when I'm by myself.* *Green Harmony*

CHAPTER 7

ENP, Quick Silver: Masters of Exercise Disguise

ENTP: Dominant Extraverted Intuition with Auxiliary Introverted Thinking
ENFP: Dominant Extraverted Intuition with Auxiliary Introverted Feeling

Energized by new ideas and possibilities, they're ready to reset their sights to embrace novel concepts and respond to a world of opportunities. No color could represent this lively type better than Silver. It's the color of mercury, shiny, fluid, and changeable.

Have you ever tried to gather up a mercury spill? Just when you think you have it cornered, it changes direction and surges down a different path. This mercurial quality helps make Silvers an exciting type, intrigued by patterns all around them, fascinated by the synergies in their worldview.

Ever-changing and always reinventing themselves, Silvers find there's little that doesn't interest them. They're quick to see connections and build on ideas. Expect them to be on the cutting edge and open to learning and exploring.

Silvers are typically busy people who sometimes risk becoming overwhelmed, having said *yes* to one too many fascinating invitations. They might drop back for a while to recoup and get their bearings, but before long, life fills up again.

Optimism comes naturally to Extraverted Intuitives—they trust in the world and believe their efforts will be successful. Facile and resourceful, Silvers attract opportunity, have an eye for recognizing it, and, when all lights are green, they engage it at just the right moment.

Silvers seldom worry about what might be in store—they're pretty sure something interesting, fun, and worthwhile will show up. They're good at quick planning, and once they get started, they're also quick on the execution. Ideas connect and a path takes shape.

Silvers pack so much into their day that convenience is a necessity. Without it, they wouldn't be able to accomplish all they set out to do. Their energy and productivity come from the excitement of new ideas and in connecting with others around those ideas. Silvers enjoy being with people who share their enthusiasm and can contribute to their projects and activities.

Exercise for its own sake is too boring for these "big picture" people. It's best when wrapped in the guise of something else, such as a challenge, adventure, exploration, or contest. Silvers may also choose to participate when physical activity is seen as a way of meeting and connecting with others. They enjoy having reasons to spend time with other people, and exercise, sports, and physical activity can fill the bill.

MOTIVATION, APPROACH, FOCUS

Of all the color types, Silvers are the most resistant to simplistic exercise—or simplistic anything. With Extraverted Intuition in the lead, they can too easily lose sensitivity to the needs of their bodies. But their ability to make connections means that the promise of increasing vitality and decreasing health threats can inspire them to bring exercise back into the picture. Silvers say the thought of being sick is unsettling; staying healthy means they can remain busy and engaged. The connection between exercise and health motivates them to be physically active as an investment in their future.

For Silvers with active friends and family, physical activity can become an operating principle in their lives. They talk of the physically active life with enthusiasm and gusto, but the momentum begins when Silvers find exercise options they can weave into the matrix of their busy days.

It's not unusual for Silvers to be "extreme exercisers," organizing much of their work, social, and family life around exercise or training for an event. When so much of life is organized around physical activity, positive momentum overpowers physical resistance. They rarely miss a day of their routine, even when it's piled on top of an already full schedule.

Laurie, a Silver with Harmony, is a personal coach. She found the perfect synergy between exercise and the rest of

---

If I had the chance, I would try almost anything, although I would not try anything too serious, too messy, or where there was no view.

—Hanna, Silver with Harmony

her life when she began joining clients out on the running path. "I started coaching people while running with them," she said. "I hardly notice that I'm exercising when I'm out there coaching clients." If she runs alone, her iPod makes it possible. "When I have to run on my own, I always listen to music—actually the radio, because when the DJs are chatting, I feel like I have company. When I skate on the canal in my hometown, Toronto, I put on my Walkman and totally enjoy being out there."

Convenience is a must, and the more decision points Silvers must navigate, the less appealing exercise becomes. Whether they belong to a gym, practice yoga or Tai Chi, bike, or run in the park, Silvers don't want to spend too much time in transition, nor do they want to fuss in the process. Their schedules are tight, time is valuable, and they want to keep their options open for interesting things that might come up.

Convenience, after all, relates to flow—moving from one activity to another with little effort—much the way Silvers connect ideas. Interruption of the flow is de-motivating, providing a reason to stop exercising, so too many stops and starts are a serious obstacle. For this reason, strength training, with its constant need to adjust weights, is irritating for most Silvers. As Marget, a Silver with Efficiency, described her reaction, "It drives me insane to adjust weight equipment. I just want to hop from machine to machine." Similarly, Pat, a Silver with Harmony and marathoner, rarely stops for water during a race. As she said, every time she stops, she'd have to decide to start again.

Siri, a yoga-loving Silver with Efficiency, keeps schedules for five or six yoga studios handy in her pocketbook. A full-time healthcare consultant and mother of two, she describes herself as "always on the fly." Whenever her busy day opens up, she consults the yoga schedules for a class that's close and convenient. In contrast to other color types that require familiarity with a facility and who develop a devotion to one teacher, what works for Siri is being able to slip a yoga practice into her schedule when it's convenient.

Most Silvers who exercise regularly fall into one of two categories: *Make it Central* or *Keep it Simple*. When physical activity takes on a *Central* role, they ride the momentum and go at it with enthusiasm, intensity, and focus—no holds barred. On the other hand, the *Keep it Simple* Silvers find exercise success by keeping activities uncomplicated, unremarkable, and easy to accomplish.

For the *Make it Central* Silvers, it's appealing to have several layers of accomplishment and enjoyment that serve to disguise pure exercise. This might include engaging in some aspect of physical activity—perhaps learning a new skill—that provides a challenge as well as including an opportunity to connect with others; this combination lets Silvers build momentum.

Penny, Silver with Efficiency, a skier, biker, and all-around athlete, gravitates to athletic friends and spends most weekends in one active pursuit or another. Physical activity is at the center of her social and family life. During the summer, Penny regularly rides with a Wednesday night biking group, delighting in keeping up with the fastest members and riding down the road at thirty-two-plus miles an hour. Her four- and five-year-olds are well on their way to becoming excellent skiers. At the age of fifty, her husband is a competitive skier. Physical activity is an important way for this family to enjoy time together.

For the *Keep it Simple* Silvers, on the other hand, the purpose of physical activity is for health and fitness. They exercise in response to their internal logic and values, in exchange for the benefits. Their aim is for health, weight management, and perhaps improved sleep.

The *Keep it Simple* Silvers, often pulled in so many directions, report that regular exercise makes them feel more balanced and in control of their lives. Exercise serves as the operating principle that brings disparate elements together and helps them gain confidence that they can deal with what comes next. The exercise itself could be a regular walk, bike ride, or jog from their home—or a yoga practice at a studio nearby. Without convenience, however, the activity is unlikely to happen.

Keep it Simple Silvers—especially Silvers with Efficiency—can sometimes become rigid in their programs, in contrast to the flexible approach they apply to the rest of

---

When I miss a few days in a row of exercise, there's a big part of me that feels like if I never exercised again I'd be happy. I make sure to get right back to the routine so I don't give in to those feelings.

—Emma, Silver with Efficiency

their lives. They may be convinced (and it's probably true) that if they deviate from their routine—or try to improve on it and change it—it will all fall apart.

Several Silvers have described their success at treating exercise as an appointment. Hanna, a Silver with Harmony, said "It's a conscious act of will." With this approach, *Keep it Simple* Silvers are not dependent on others. They initiate and complete their regular exercise sessions—often alone.

ENVIRONMENT AND PERSONAL CONNECTIONS

As stated earlier, Silvers' preferred environment for exercise is based on convenience and flexibility. When things get too structured, with too many steps intervening between the decision to exercise and actually doing it, the activity becomes less appealing and stands to lose out to other interests. They prefer to get their exercise outdoors, which can be more convenient than getting themselves to a class or the gym.

Silvers' many interests are engaged through variety, which also wards off boredom. Patrick, a Silver with Efficiency, advises: "Try to find three or four venues so you can rotate."

Silvers need their exercise in disguise. They're not exercising, they're doing Tai Chi, or playing tennis. They are not lifting weights, they're moving rocks from the garden. It's not about the Pilates class, it's about going out to lunch with classmates after the session. In that case, the real hook is socializing, not Pilates.

Connecting with people around training programs—possibly taking the lead in setting up their program and training schedule—helps keep the activity central and Silver's commitment high. Rachelle, a Silver with Harmony, said, "I commit to others. We always e-mail each other the night before to see who is running the next day so no one has to run alone. If I say I'm going to run, then I show up. I don't bail out on the people I've committed to. I notice if I leave it as a 'maybe,' if the weather is too cold or something else comes up, I'm likely to bail."

Hamilton, at age seventy-five, loves training for the 100-yard dash with a group of other seniors at the local university track-and-field facility. Training with people he respects and enjoys and traveling to track meets throughout the country is fun and provides the opportunity to push toward higher and higher limits—a great goal for Silvers with Efficiency, who are always striving to expand their reach.

SILVERS WITH EFFICIENCY (ENTP)

Silvers with Efficiency aren't just big picture people—they get their view from 35,000 feet. They're constantly using their broad scope to make new connections and imagine new possibilities, at a pace that might dizzy other types.

Silvers with Efficiency love to team with and learn from others, and there's little that doesn't interest them. Welcoming all perspectives, always pleased to add more information into the mix, they're respectful of others' viewpoints. They love verbal banter and can take either side of an argument.

With their fast-paced minds and penchant for complexity, there's virtually nothing that a Silver with Efficiency can't connect with, improve on, and raise to a higher level—including exercise. For many Silvers with Efficiency, it doesn't occur to them to do anything in an ordinary way.

Passing the time quickly is an important element for fast-paced Silvers with Efficiency. Attention on something more interesting (and just about everything is more interesting than pure exercise) helps, as long as it doesn't compete with and gain their total attention. For instance, if they get too engrossed in a TV program while lifting weights, they might put down the dumbbells and just watch the news. Finding the right amount of distraction can be a challenge.

Exercising with others gives Silvers with Efficiency an additional layer to focus on, passing the time more quickly. Whether it's the accountability of a group training session, walking or biking with a friend, or swimming alongside someone in the next lane, having other people around keeps the energy and focus levels up.

Silvers with Efficiency are particularly intrigued by yoga and report that it fully engages them. Harris enjoys it because it's a vigorous workout that doesn't seem like exercise. He likes the theory behind yoga, and as he describes it, "the practice gives me a place to put my brain." He notes, "I wouldn't like it if it didn't have the mental dimension. It's interesting to learn, for instance, that the only way to stretch your hamstrings is to engage your quads."

Silvers can combine exercise with their natural curiosity to add another layer of accomplishment (the more the better, say Silvers with Efficiency). A walking meeting with colleagues can provide the double benefit of work and exercise. Mary, a Silver with Efficiency and power company executive, had a successful dog walking business as a young teenager. As she described it,

"It gave me a built-in excuse to be outside for hours." Her type's entrepreneurial nature kicked in early. As she notes twenty years later, "It was one of the best jobs of my life."

Jess organized a bike ride across the country with a group of fellow graduates from Wharton. The biking was incredible, but she was hooked by the secondary benefits. Putting together a plan, she learned bike routes, investigated weather, updated friends by e-mail, and researched great places to stay and see. She saw America not by the highways, but the byways, and reaped great physical exercise in the process.

Once they begin exercising, Silvers with Efficiency find interruption of their momentum and flow discouraging. Packing a gym bag, driving to the gym, and changing clothes in the locker room all fly in the face of efficient Silver goals; they break the momentum and remind them that there are more interesting things to do than exercise.

With their expansive natures, Silvers with Efficiency enjoy being outside. It calms them and releases some of the pressure that can build up internally. It also can provide much needed alone time to reflect, analyze information, and quietly sift through the many opportunities that come their way.

SILVERS WITH HARMONY (ENFP)

While the hallmark of Silvers with Efficiency is intense engagement, for Silvers with Harmony it's fun engagement. Enjoyment is the key for them, regardless of the activity—and fun usually includes other people. This type is optimistic, with playful personalities that naturally seek out meaningful activities that align with their closely-held values.

Said Laurie, a Silver with Harmony, "I'm definitely not always having fun when I exercise, but if it's not fun, it quickly gets dropped for something else." But it's not as easy as it looks. People who watch Silvers with Harmony exercising think they are having the "time of their life" and envy how easy it is for them to engage in physical activity. What they don't see is the effort this type makes to trick themselves into that exercise.

Exercise for Silvers with Harmony is not about the exercise—it's the alternative purpose that's the hook that keeps them coming back. For example, they do yoga for spiritual integration, run outdoors for the love and appreciation of nature, condition to be in top form to play tennis with business colleagues, or cross-country ski because they love to be in the mountains with friends.

Silvers with Harmony readily make the body/mind/spirit connection. For many of them, physical activity supports and connects them to their spiritual side. The "higher limits" they are trying to reach through exercise intrigue and motivate them.

When they are fitness instructors—and they frequently are—Silvers with Harmony are high energy and will do all they can to make the class fun and varied. Don't expect the same routine in the next session—that would be too boring.

Silvers with Harmony enjoy plenty of diversity and variety in exercise. With their steep learning curve and love of exploring, they are challenged by new and fun activities. As Rachelle told me, "I can do anything, as long as it's not the only thing I do."

Often, diversity takes the form of cycling through activities. For instance, they might do Bikram yoga and throw themselves into it—attending five classes a week for a year, perhaps even becoming a Bikram yoga teacher. But after a while, bored with Bikram, they become intrigued with training for a weight lifting contest. Next, they might join a group preparing for a triathlon.

For Silvers with Harmony, the outdoors is their playground. Being under blue skies, with clean air, fresh snow, or swaying palm trees, provides all the elements Silvers with Harmony need to get active.

MEET THE SILVERS

Jessica, Silver with Efficiency (ENTP)

Fast moving and fast talking, Jessica graduated from Dartmouth at age 21 and went directly to her first job in Russia. To land the position, she used her dominant Perceiving process to draw all sorts of connections and follow multiple avenues in pursuit of an offer. She researched Russian companies, contacted U.S. businesses that maintain offices in Russia, networked with friends and the parents of friends, and contacted whoever seemed likely to provide a lead.

As a former career counselor, I was curious whether she worked with the outstanding Career Services office at Dartmouth. "No, it never occurred to me," Jess said. With so many new avenues and connections to attract her attention, she didn't notice the old familiar resources at her elbow—a typical Silver way to be.

Now with a Wharton MBA to her credit and her career solidly in place, Jess still makes ample time in her schedule to train for athletic competitions—anything from a swim across the Chesapeake River, a triathlon at Lake Placid, or the Marine Marathon in Washington, D.C.

Much of Jess's social life centers on physical activity. With exercise woven throughout her day, she enjoys a level of positive momentum that overpowers any resistance. When exercise takes this kind of central role in Silvers' lives, the activity itself becomes an organizing principle around which their schedules revolve. As Jess said, "I do some activity every day. I rarely miss a day. A regular person's schedule would not permit it—but I make it happen."

For Silvers, living in a culture that supports exercise—or better yet, one designed for it—creates an activity flow that is rewarding and self-sustaining. How fitting that Jess met her fiancé at a running club and he proposed to her on a run!

Did you ever notice someone at the gym on the next treadmill with a towel covering the electronic readouts? Or have you wondered why some people enjoy wearing a heart rate monitor while others hate it? Jessica expressed what many Silvers know: It all has to do with flow.

"I dislike wearing a monitor," Jess said. "I don't like to know whether I'm pushing myself or not. Clocks constrain and limit; they're confining measurements. For me,

exercise is about making the time pass quickly," Jess said. "I love it, but I want to get on with the rest of my day."

Leo, Silver with Efficiency (ENTP)

Leo is an entrepreneur and founder of a large chain of quick service restaurants. At the age of sixty-two, he's actively involved as a director on nine boards—four of which he chairs. A man of many interests, he can speak with authority on varied topics, including wine, history, and literature, which are much more fun to contemplate than exercise. His wide-ranging knowledge coupled with his outstanding analytical skills make him an engaging conversationalist.

A Silver with Efficiency, Leo explained why he doesn't belong to a gym. "There are too many steps involved," he said. "You have to pack your bag, drive to the gym, change into gym clothes, shower after working out, change back into work clothes—it's a lot of wasted effort, and I wouldn't do it."

Leo prefers to roll out of bed, take a walk or a bike ride, then clean up once before launching into the rest of his day. "I'm more inclined to exercise if it's easy to start and there's no commitment or plan," he said. "If I take a walk and the weather is nice, I can walk for a long time. If the weather is not so nice—I can turn around. There's no burden or obligation."

"The easiest thing for me is walking and talking with someone else," Leo said. "The time goes by quickly. I don't even think of it as exercise. There's no resistance to overcome."

Leo has developed considerable insight into his own character, which comes into play when he's devising ways to keep physical activity in his life. "It's always a balance whether the obligation outweighs my resistance to the obligation," he said. "I don't like to be dictated to, even by myself."

There's very little exercise that Leo enjoys for its own sake; he does it for specific reasons. "I know it's good for my health, and I sleep better," he said. And he recognizes which elements make it more likely that he'll keep it up.

"The evidence was compelling for me to begin a program of weight training—but I really resisted it," he remembered. "My wife weight-trained at home and the weights had already been conveniently set up. She bugged me to use them, but I continued to resist. Finally, she made it so easy that I agreed."

She engaged a personal trainer to come to their home. "My wife chose someone she knew I would like, who would be very effi-cient," Leo said. He wanted a routine that would take no more than twenty minutes. And he wanted it simple.

"The trainer taught me a routine that hit all major muscle groups as efficiently as possible," he said. Yet, learning the routine proved a considerable challenge. "It was alien to my experience," Leo recalled. "No TV news, door closed. The process required a complete personal commitment." The weights and a bench are located in his office, and Leo uses them several times a week. "I'm on automatic pilot now. It doesn't require so much focused attention. I can even do sets in between e-mails!"

Ernie, Silver with Harmony (ENFP)

Ernie smiles when he talks about his active life. Six foot three, handsome, and notice-ably fit, he is the president of a large real estate company. Ernie is a member of a number of non-profit boards, and is a well-known leader in his community. The main-stay of his physical life is his dedication to Tai Chi. For the past fifteen years, he's been practicing it every morning for thirty to sixty minutes, always outdoors, even during the cold of a Northeast winter.

"When I practice Tai Chi, I take in every conceivable natural element around me,"

Ernie said. "For 365 days a year, I see the seasons change; I see the same squirrels; I see the blossoms grow into flowers; the leaves come out, then die, and then go through the same process all over again. I see the rain, the sun, the darkness, the brightness. I'm totally engaged with everything that is going on around me. And I'm trying to meditate through it, creating energy."

Tai Chi provides him with both an opportunity to get outdoors and a spiritual component, with a beauty and flow all its own. But that's just the beginning. Ernie also engages in activities that include Astanga and Bikram yoga, competitive sailing, swimming, water skiing, tennis, golf, and downhill skiing.

However, none of these activities is about exercise for its own sake. Ernie has a word for them: "They're *fun,* and they provide a nice combination of activities in my life," he said. His activity list breaks down according to various dimensions of his life. Skiing, tennis, and golf are social. "They're enjoyable and I do them with other people. It's beautiful being outside. And I love skiing with my daughter."

Sailing and water sports are social, but they also provide good physical and mental workouts. "In the summer, I water-ski and sail like crazy. I race and find it freeing."

Ernie talked about sailing as a meditation. "You cannot sail well without finding your connection to nature. The simple variations on the theme of wind movement can win or lose you a race. The tides, the waves, the wind, the sun create thermals. Circumstances can become dangerous, or be absolutely calm. Nature on the water has many personalities. You don't fight it; you become it. Work with it and use it to propel you."

Ernie also goes to several Bikram yoga classes a week. "I like the intensity of doing ninety minutes in heat. If I do it in heat, my muscles don't hurt the next day. Sweating is very cathartic and detoxifying. I get a natural high that lasts for a day. I also do stretching at home. I don't do weights because the yoga and Tai Chi take care of that."

At the end of our interview, I asked Ernie if he was satisfied with what he is doing. "Oh yes! But other people think I'm crazy."

Susanne, Silver with Harmony (ENFP)

Running provides just the right combination of healthy exercise and fun for Susanne. It lets her connect with people and explore her world. She keeps it new by learning about her body's abilities and challenging herself to ever-higher goals.

Susanne lives in New York City, where

she began running shortly after she moved there from Switzerland. She joined the New York Road Runners Club, and it became the core of her friendship network.

Susanne integrates elements of her running routine and its discipline into other areas of her life. "Now I want to run smarter—do more interval training," she said. "I've also become a vegetarian, and several other runners and I are experimenting with food."

Running provides a nice balance to Susanne's busy life as a human resources director. In addition to running with her

---

A SILVER WITH EFFICIENCY DESCRIBES THE ULTIMATE GYM EXPERIENCE

I love working out at my fitness club because of the extraordinary quality of everything they do, from making sure every guest locker is stocked with hangers for my clothes, to continuously renewing the supply of towels and soaps. Everything is in place and well cared for.

All of the added services—dry cleaning, hair salon and spa, restaurants—are up to the same standard. I'm greeted with a smile at the entrance, and there's always a trainer to happily explain new gym equipment. With 11,000 members, and a live jazz band that plays nightly, the club is active and welcoming. There's a palpable sense of community.

And the food! The club has two restaurants and a prepared-food shop that serve some of the healthiest, most delicious, and well-priced food in town. I arrive at the gym after work, attend a great class, and perhaps do some cardio on the tread climber before taking a leisurely steam, hot tub, or sauna. I shower and dress and pick up dinner in the Grill or at the prepared food counter, then drive home. Between the live jazz band, bustling atmosphere, attractive people, and excellent dinner, I feel like I've had an evening out! I thoroughly enjoy working out at a place that offers so much.

group, she also does it solo. As she said, "Running alone is my introverted time. I plan my day, pre-write papers, memorize stuff. It clears my mind."

Susanne is now a running coach for her community. Coaching enables her to support others in reaching their goals, which provides an additional layer of meaning to the sport.

All of Susanne's training takes place outdoors. Even during New York winters, she runs outside, saying treadmills and indoor gyms are too confining. To keep running interesting, each year she trains for several marathons that take place in different parts of the United States. "It's a great way to see the country, and our group always stays in very nice hotels and has a great time," she said.

I asked Susanne for her recommendation for Silvers with Harmony who want to start exercising. She would approach them by inviting them out into the natural world. She knows for Silvers with Harmony, the route to a physically active life is to enjoy what they do and learn about their world. Exercise is the peripheral benefit. "It's important to take it out of the context of exercise. I'd ask them to join me in finding something interesting—let's explore and talk."

FAVORITE ACTIVITIES

Biking: A favorite Silver activity, it's a way to enjoy the outdoors, whether with friends or alone. Biking is also convenient: it can start from the front door, or, if traveling with a bike, from almost anywhere. A bike ride can be peaceful and at the same time challenging. It also offers the additional opportunity to explore.

Cardiovascular machines and fitness classes: Silvers are inclined to use fitness centers that provide a combination of variety, interest, and convenience. They enjoy having options and might keep their energy up by rotating through the various cardio machines. A menu of drop-in fitness classes provides additional opportunities, and a well-trained and interested staff is noted and appreciated.

Dancing: With their flare for drama and love of performance and self-expression, Silvers enjoy many types of dance: Salsa, folk, flamingo, swing, and ballroom. Silvers with Efficiency often enjoy competitive ballroom dancing, with the opportunity it provides to travel to competitions.

Hiking: Hiking offers opportunities for Silvers to explore and connect with others.

The momentum of a group or family hike can keep the interest level high, increasing the likelihood of making it to the top of the mountain.

Running: This activity provides the biggest bang for the buck, an important consideration for Silvers. With few equipment requirements other than a pair of running shoes, this is one of the most convenient of all sports. Meeting and training with others is a great way for Silvers to socialize and keep the momentum up.

Skiing: In snowy climates, skiing provides great exercise and a wonderful opportunity to explore. Silvers especially gravitate toward Nordic skiing, but also can enjoy downhill skiing, as long as lift lines are not too long. It's a fun activity to share with others.

Yoga and Tai Chi: Silvers gravitate toward yoga and Tai Chi for the body/mind/spirit connections. These disciplines provide intellectual and spiritual interest while stressing balance and peacefulness, and can also provide an ongoing challenge.

ROADBLOCKS AND TIPS

Roadblocks

- Ideas and mental stimulation monopolize attention
- Ignoring the body
- Viewing exercise as boring and a cause of suffering
- Inconvenience

Top 10 Tips

1. It's not about exercise. Disguise exercise within something more appealing than pure exercise—something else that's interesting, enjoyable, and engaging.
2. Choose activities that will provide an opportunity to explore and learn something new, creating many levels and layers of achievement and interest. Exercise can take you to new and different places

I'm streaky about going to the gym. I'll go consistently for a month, then nothing for the next two months. I'll work out most when there's a reason, such as basketball season or before going to the beach.

—Russ, Silver with Efficiency

and provide experiences you can't get any other way. Satisfy your natural curiosity by learning about the physiology of the body, or perhaps achieving peace through experiencing the body/mind/spirit connection.

3. Just begin and see where it takes you. Don't wait until you can do it at the highest level, or until conditions are otherwise "perfect." Once you're working out, you're more likely to continue. For instance, if you're lifting weights, start with what's easiest and most enjoyable, not the most difficult.

4. Teach fitness. What better way to keep exercise in your life? Your inclination toward variety and a high-energy approach will appeal to others and keep you moving.

5. Coordinate and be accountable to others to counter the "Do I feel like it?" tendency. Keep up with calls and e-mail interaction prior to getting together. Working out with others raises your level of performance and is more fun. A get-together afterwards sweetens the deal.

6. Monitor progress and chart achievement at long intervals. Frequent monitoring (readouts on cardiovascular equipment, heart rate monitors, and clocks) can be discouraging.

7. To balance your busy and interactive life, build in some alone exercise time, for planning and reflection. This should be repetitive in nature (walking, running, biking) and not require focused attention.

8. Keep transition processes minimal and decision points few. Go to the gym in workout clothes to avoid "wasted" time in the locker room. Don't get sidetracked along the way. Checking e-mail, starting to read an article, or beginning a conversation on the way out the door means you'll need to decide again to exercise.

9. Convenience is a priority. Choose activities that can be easily accessed, and keep equipment handy. If you have to search for your sneakers, your motivation could flag.

10. Look for fast-paced dance or fitness classes that are fun and can easily be slipped into the day.

SILVER WORDS

Competency, convenience, creativity, distractions, efficiency, energy, enjoyment, flow, fun, health, innovation, momentum, optimism, person connections, spontaneity, unscripted

Silvers at a Glance—Quick Silver: Masters of Exercise Disguise

ENTP: Silver Efficiency—Dominant Extraverted Intuition with Auxiliary Introverted Thinking

ENFP: Silver Harmony—Dominant Extraverted Intuition with Auxiliary Introverted Feeling

Overall Qualities	Silvers wrap exercise in a disguise, as the idea of pure exercise is unappealing; an alternative purpose keeps them engaged. Silvers enjoy activities that are convenient, requiring minimal process and planning. Silvers are attracted to new ideas and possibilities and activities with others. They enjoy variety and tend to cycle through fitness passions. Or, they might avoid the temptation of novelty and keep their exercise program routine and simple.
Motivation:	• Threats to health and well being • Connections with people and exploring the world • Fun and enjoyment—exercise as a peripheral benefit • Physical activity benefits mind/body/spirit
Approach:	• Create multiple layers of achievement and experience • Seek variety—will try novel or "cutting edge" activities • Ride positive momentum from activity/people, or keep routine simple • Minimize process and decision points

Focus:	• Direct attention to something more enjoyable than exercise • Energized by the body/mind/spirit connection • Enjoy learning something new • Watch television when engaged in repetitious cardio activities
Environments:	• Convenient—minimal steps to get going • Outdoors preferred—releases internal pressure • Gym activities that require little advanced planning
Interpersonal Connections:	• Coordinating/exercising with others creates accountability • Physical activities with others is fun • Use exercise as alone time for planning and reflection
Sample Quotes:	*I want to get the biggest bang for my buck. That means the least time and the most benefit. It drives me insane to adjust weight equipment. I just want to jump from machine to machine. I want a trainer who understands the body and can explain it to me. It is important that he/she be competent.* *Silver Efficiency* *When I practice Tai Chi outside, it is not only exercise, but a meditation. I can't do it without taking in every conceivable natural piece around me. I see the squirrels, the birds, and the blossoms. I'm totally engrossed in everything that is going on around me and I'm trying to meditate through it while creating energy.* *Silver Harmony*

CHAPTER 8

INP, Saffron Seeking: Making Workouts into Play

INTP: Dominant Introverted Thinking with Auxiliary Extraverted Intuition
INFP: Dominant Introverted Feeling with Auxiliary Extraverted Intuition

Evocative of a rare and valuable spice from India, or the colored robes worn by Buddhist monks, this type is exemplified by the phrase "still waters run deep." Saffron is a burnt orange hue that commands attention with its intensity, but in a warm and comfortable way. There is no glitz or extravagance involved.

Similar to Silvers, Saffrons are easygoing and casual, and their lifestyles follow that lead. They're attracted by comfortable clothes, lots of fresh air, and easy access to exercise that requires minimal process or advance planning.

Some types dedicate themselves to organizing and locking in activities ahead of time, but not Saffrons. Keeping plans to a minimum provides more opportunities to enjoy the kick they get when life hands them the unexpected. For them, serendipity provides an extra measure of enjoyment and fun.

Saffrons don't trudge through life, they are ready to grasp it and respond to opportunities as they emerge. Whether it's going for a run on a windy afternoon, Salsa dancing, or joining a ski team at the urging of a friend, they prefer minimal structure, keeping things casual and flexible. Knowing they'll be free to make changes when an activity gets tedious can be reassuring.

But don't be fooled by their relaxed outward demeanor. Inwardly, Saffrons can be intense. With a challenge in front of them, they apply themselves to the task with quiet commitment. Competitive—with themselves more than with others—Saffrons are engaged by setting difficult and often physically demanding goals and then proceeding to accomplish them. Physical pursuits are in fact a great balance to their intensity, providing a cleansing relief from constant inner analysis, debate, and searching.

Independent, and often perfectionists, they're drawn to activities that require a high level of performance. Boredom can be a concern for them. Saffrons find satisfaction and often a sense of spiritual involvement (especially Saffrons with Harmony) in physical pursuits that push them to higher levels. Flow and rhythm are essential in these pursuits.

Don't try to pin Saffrons down before they're ready. Holding off on final decisions supports their need for flexibility. Unresponsive to coercion, they make choices based on internal analysis (Saffrons with Efficiency) or their own values (Saffrons with Harmony). They might politely listen to a doctor's rehab suggestions after surgery, but they'll comply only if the regimen makes sense based on their personal logic and principles. They'll bring their intellect to bear, appreciating professional viewpoints, but weighing in with their own thoughts on a subject.

MOTIVATION, APPROACH, FOCUS

For Saffrons to maintain physical activity, they must find in it elements of challenge, fun, freedom, and flow. Without this combination, it's difficult for Saffrons to garner the necessary energy and commitment for physical activity; they can find so many other interesting pursuits to occupy their time. Whereas Silvers have wide and varied interests and can become engaged in almost any type of activity, Saffrons have more specific needs and requirements.

Saffrons look for outlets that require a measure of skill and effort, often with a touch of novelty thrown in. Exercise should be fun, but it's the challenge that provides the appeal. Because they're easily bored, this becomes an issue with typical forms of routine exercise.

Though this type appreciates being physically active, imposed routines and schedules limit Saffrons' flexibility to engage on their own terms and soon become burdens that inhibit rather than encourage them to continue with an activity. However, when they find a physical pursuit that resonates with them, Saffrons can be totally engaged and throw themselves into it with great energy.

I've found the perfect exercise. I can exercise, meditate, and relax all at the same time. Gazing at the black line on the bottom of the pool when I swim laps, I can sort out my life.

—Jon, Saffron with Harmony

As with Silvers, convenience is another important consideration—most say it's essential—for making physical activity appealing to Saffrons. Every step they must take on the way to exercising is another opportunity to get off track, so the fewer decision points between the idea and its execution, the better. The bike, inaccessible because it's hanging too high in the garage, could discourage a Saffron from taking a ride. But the real deal breaker is the addition of a back tire that needs pumping. The opportunity is lost.

By its very nature, music helps keep the flow going and draws Saffrons in. With iPod in hand, a Saffron described the importance of music to him: "It's always been the one thing I like to have with me when I'm working out," he said. "Without music, it's twice as hard."

Being open-ended and oriented toward new opportunities, Saffrons easily connect and respond to creative ideas and novel choices that come their way. Unlike Whites, who envision their exercise ahead of time and consider planning to be part of the process and the enjoyment, Saffrons love the good fortune of getting an invitation (from nature or another person) that they can respond to immediately. They like nothing better than taking advantage of the moment when a new weather system moves in and the hills are covered with snow for skiing, or when ocean waves are perfect for surfing. For them, spontaneity is part of the fun.

ENVIRONMENT AND PERSONAL CONNECTIONS

Saffrons enjoy exercising alone—*and* with others. If running is their exercise of choice, they may turn up the iPod and spend time with their thoughts or daydreaming. At other times, they might enjoy running with someone else, exchanging a few words rather than getting into an involved discussion.

Erik, a Saffron with Efficiency, often "picks up" with people he encounters on the bike path. "I see someone I want to run

There's a wonderful freedom about dance. I loved the leap, reaching the point where you're weightless. It's amazing how your body feels physically.

—Kathy, Saffron with Harmony

with and say, 'Hey, can I join you?' When I'm not in great shape, it's easier to run with another person. No one has ever said no. A few weeks ago I was having difficulty running and I picked up the cross-country coach from a local college. It helped—it was easier to run with him than by myself. I guess running with another person gets me out of my head."

Bill, a Saffron with Efficiency and boulderer, agrees. When he's engaged in his sport (a style of rock climbing without the use of ropes or safety equipment), he's fully focused. "You're living in the moment," he said. "I don't think about anything but that very next move."

It's not unusual to see Saffrons training for a marathon with a family member or friend, but this won't happen if there's much to-do about dates and schedules ahead of time. It's got to be convenient and relaxed.

A Saffron might also enjoy running with a colleague from work, meeting seamlessly at lunchtime to exercise together. Proximity and ease of scheduling make it happen— remember, convenience for this type is a must. Because Saffrons rarely consider themselves part of a group, they deal better with a few like-minded people, rather than an organized gathering. Note the difference with Silvers, who are energized by groups.

With their preference for freedom and flow, Saffrons typically choose the outdoors for cardio activities over those in gyms and clubs. Kathy, a Saffron with Harmony, lives in a retirement community surrounded by lush woods and walking paths where she gets regular exercise walking her dog, Hermes. She recalls the day the community's wellness coordinator showed her around the gym and fitness center with its stationary bikes, treadmills, and elliptical machines. Appreciating the facility but finding it joyless, Kathy said amiably, "I don't do machines."

Responding to challenges and indulging their penchant for novelty and play, Saffrons like games that require skill or strategy, or activities that hold some meaning for them.

Among all the Introverted color types (Blues, Greens, Saffrons, and Whites), it is Saffrons who most often report enjoying the experience of exercising in the company of others. However, note that the interaction cannot be demanding or confining. Going out for a run or hike with the family, dogs included, works well. They find solitary exercise alongside other people to be very satisfying.

SAFFRONS WITH EFFICIENCY (INTP)

Outwardly casual, Saffrons with Efficiency are inwardly intense, demanding, and precise. They are engaged in a never-ending internal analysis, which may be why play is so important to them. When they're physically engaged, they can turn off their analytical mind and focus on something with an element of fun to it, whether a substantial challenge like bouldering or something simpler, such as a run on a beautiful day or a game of Ultimate Frisbee.

Exercise, then, is a welcome relief for this type, providing much-needed balance. Although stress management is one of the great benefits of exercise for all types, for this color type it's of primary importance. Exercise provides an opportunity to, as some have described it, "sort things out, take time to think about things and not react to them." As one Saffron with Efficiency put it, "I can go into exercise with something bugging me and leave like it's been handled."

"When I don't work out for a week, I feel sluggish, depressed, and stressed out," said Trent, who talked about moving from Los Angeles back to his home in Washington, D.C. "When I moved back from L.A., it was a very stressful time. I asked myself what was the most constructive thing I could do. Working out gave me a purpose, a direction, a goal. It was something that I could accomplish."

Saffrons with Efficiency are relentlessly logical. With internal analysis as an ongoing and constant process, it makes sense that a simple stroll on their own is not a particularly appealing exercise option. They need more to focus on. And focus they do, at least for a time. Typically, Saffrons with Efficiency find themselves powerfully committed to exercise for a period, and then they lose interest or become bored and stop.

Exercising with others provides an interesting perk for this color type. A shared activity brings a welcome opportunity to

[INTPs] are motivated by intellectual and complex challenge. The tougher the problem, the greater the interest

—Roger Pearman, *You, Being More Effective in Your MBTI Type* (2005)

spend time with people without the need to engage in small talk, which is often difficult to sustain. With their dominant Introverted Thinking, they place a high premium on logic and analysis. It's not surprising that generating or participating in small talk with no particular purpose can be uncomfortable for them.

The intensity of a good challenge keeps Saffrons with Efficiency solidly engaged. If the activity is also enjoyable enough to appeal to their playful side, a Saffron is hooked—at least for a while.

SAFFRONS WITH HARMONY (INFP)

There is no type whose exercise choices exemplify the concept of "different strokes for different folks" more than Saffron with Harmony. Guided by heartfelt values, they are passionate about everything they do. Their convictions are at the core of their decisions, and values bring meaning to their lives. As one Saffron with Harmony

told me: "I don't know how I could decide anything if it wasn't for values." Members of this color type cherish their time, and they make careful choices for how they'll spend it. They'd rather do nothing than waste time on something they dislike.

Saffrons with Harmony hold self-expression close to their hearts; they are drawn to exercise with an element of fun and creativity. Hooked by movement that flows, many Saffrons with Harmony who become fitness instructors are in fact former dancers; they transition their love of fluid movement to the world of fitness.

Because values are so individualized for these dominant Introverted Feeling types, Saffrons with Harmony show the greatest diversity in their choice of exercise. One college president goes all out three times a day—a morning run, a noon swim, and an evening run. My Saffron-with-Harmony sister-in-law loves tap dancing and walking. As for a technical writer, downhill freestyle ski racing is her passion.

I have joined running and bicycling groups before and quickly un- joined them. They don't turn me off, but I feel I don't fit in so I drop out.

—Anastasia, Saffron with Harmony

Their chosen activities engage and focus these Saffrons, providing opportunities for individual expression through movement. Although their favored activities are as different as the individuals in this type, look closely and you'll find a common thread. What they share is the way they use the flow of exercise as a means of self-expression—movement expressing the self without speech. The flow is fundamental. This may explain why dance—all manner of dance—is so inviting.

As fond as they are of fluid movement, Saffrons with Harmony can be highly competitive in physical activity. When this is the case, it's the competition that creates the fun. As one Saffron with Harmony described it: "It gives me something to chase after."

MEET THE SAFFRONS

Karen, Saffron with Efficiency (INTP)

Karen is twenty-five years old and owns seven bikes, a couple of which can be found in the back of her station wagon at any particular time. Blonde, fit, and low-key, Karen is partial to T-shirts, jeans, and sweaters.

Karen took two years off after her first year at college to work as a bicycle mechanic and massage therapist for various profes-sional cycling teams. Now finished with her education and working part time as a massage therapist, biking and skiing are Karen's mainstay activities. "I like to go out and play," she said. "If it's not fun, it doesn't really count as exercise."

Typical of Saffrons with Efficiency, fun is fundamental, but intensity is also a hook. Karen described her enjoyment of Kung Fu: "I liked the intensity of it. And the purpose was for self-defense. I knew what the options were, and I had a fantastic instructor who was knowledgeable and pushed me hard."

Now Karen trains regularly and races downhill mountain bikes. She acknowledges a concern with boredom. "That's why I like downhill bike racing," she said. "I'm never bored."

Karen enjoys biking alone, and with others. "I usually ride by myself," she said. "When I do solo excursions, I let my mind wander. I process a lot of stuff. It's good study time. But I also enjoy riding with a couple of other people, as long as we all want to do the same thing. I've been around bike people for a while and they're usually very skills-oriented. You can learn a lot by following someone else down the trail."

Showing her efficient side, plus her desire to exercise with like-minded people, she added, "I'm not going to bike with the wrong person more than once."

Karen doesn't think about daily exercise; she envisions it in weekly chunks: "If I think daily and don't have time, I feel I've failed for that day," she explained. "I rarely exercise if I don't want to. I can make myself do it if I think about it for a purpose—like loosening up or knowing I'm going to feel better. But generally, there's nothing I do that's typical. It's pretty much what I feel like doing."

Biking is her activity of choice; maintaining fitness is a means to an end. "If I have a good base of fitness, I'm happy," Karen said. As an athlete who trains intensively, from time to time she purposely takes "mental rests" from exercise—sometimes for days, sometimes weeks. These mental rests remove the pressure to train and exercise, an important consideration for Saffrons with Efficiency, who may start to feel bogged down or exhausted from the pressure of a regimen aimed at a goal.

"I find that once I allow myself that space, I'm more motivated to go outside and play."

It's also important not to get discouraged if you're out of shape, she said: "One of the neat things about returning to exercise when you're out of shape is that you see results so quickly. Improvements come week-to-week or even day-to-day. It's incredible."

Typical of all Saffrons—Efficients and Harmonies—Karen does her cardio activities outdoors. "I go to a gym only for a particular purpose, like lifting weights," she said. "I bike outside during most of the winter, in temperatures down to twenty degrees. It feels natural to be outside. It's a comfortable place to be."

Dick, Saffron with Efficiency (INTP)

Dick is an organizational consultant living in Minneapolis. He exercises five or six times a week in a variety of activities that include biking or running in the hills of a nature area near his office, working out on an elliptical machine, and swimming at a gym.

A typical Saffron with Efficiency, Dick prefers to exercise outdoors whenever the weather permits. If that's not possible, he visits one of two gyms where he's a member—one near his office, primarily for swimming, and the other near his home, for cardio machines. Although Dick acknowledges the expense of belonging to two gyms, he loves the convenience.

"Convenience is part of the flow," he said. "I like the flexibility of being able to decide in the morning or at the end of the day what I'll do. This way I can go for a swim in the evening, or if the weather is crisp and clear, I can go for a run. I like having several different structures—it makes getting exercise more available."

Dick said he loves creating a rhythm and keeping it going. "That's why I don't like lifting weights," he said. "Changing weights for each body part—so many stops and starts. There's no flow to weight lifting, and I find it very difficult to do."

His current favorite activity is mountaineering: "I love it because it's physically demanding, and then I can rest. Part of the reason I exercise is so I can rest."

Dick, like Karen, engages in exercise that enables intense focus so he won't be bored. He lets things happen without too much structure, but puts himself in environments where things are likely to happen. Karen's bikes are in her car; Dick belongs to two fitness clubs.

Linda, Saffron with Harmony (INFP)

Linda has been running and competing in races for twenty-six years. Petite at one hundred pounds, this nurse practitioner, mother of five, and grandmother of eight, has competed in the rigorous Ironman in Hawaii each year for the past several years, regularly completing the world-renowned triathlon that consists of a 2.4-mile ocean swim, a 112-mile bike race, and a 26.2-mile run.

A triathlon is a singular and solitary pursuit, but training for it can incorporate working with others. Linda is typical of Saffrons with Harmony in this respect, avoiding regimentation where she can. She likes her training program to be planned, but flexible enough to keep an element of spontaneity. If someone suggests she come along on a bike ride, she likes to be free enough to accept the invitation.

Linda's son has been a professional triathlete. The two work in concert to keep Linda in condition; she refers to him as her "casual coach." She talks to him about her training program and he makes recommendations, but in the end, Linda devises her own routines. For one Ironman event, her son prepared a three-page program that Linda took along to Hawaii for reference, but she used her own judgment for final decisions. She appreciates expert commentary on her strategy, but she doesn't like to be told what to do.

Linda's activity choices during the entire year are broad—running, biking, cross-country skiing, swimming, yoga—but there is a common thread. All of these choices involve free-flowing movement, which is motivating for Saffrons with Harmony.

The one activity that rises above the others for Linda is running; she's passionate about it. As she describes it, running is part of the journey of her life. The language she uses when discussing her attraction to the sport—to such demanding tests of strength and will—evokes the mystical significance the activity holds for her. As she wrote for the triathlon newsletter *Masters in Motion—Dedicated to Women Master Triathletes* (Fourth Quarter 95, Vol. 3, Issue 6):

> For the past several years I've been asking myself why I continue to "do" Triathlon. Until this summer I could only sense my need to do this inwardly and could not explain myself logically to anyone. Logic cannot provide an answer.
>
> In my individual journey I both find and lose myself and then rediscover what is important to me. These journeys in the form of Triathlon, for example, cause me to repeatedly encounter challenges which I choose to meet and overcome. In life we do not always have the opportunity to choose our challenges, hopefully our efforts in Triathlon help us to respond with ever more confidence, wisdom and serenity.
>
> To race for fun, to "keep in shape," to enjoy the rush of competition, to socialize with compatriots—none of these hit the mark. Dramatic as it may sound, I know there is a profoundly meaningful phenomenon occurring deep within my soul.

Linda and other Saffrons with Harmony need a meaningful reason to focus their attention on physical activity. She finds personal significance in the effort to better herself physically and mentally while working toward a worthy goal. Running is about her life's journey, and the triathlon is a metaphor for that.

"Self-improvement is my whole life," Linda says. "I want to do what I'm passionate about."

Panio: Saffron with Harmony (INFP)

Panio finds every hook that could draw a Saffron to exercise in Tae Kwon Do, which he has practiced since he was fourteen. What appears to be a series of separate kicks, jumps, and jabs is, instead, as he describes it, "all about flow. I am attracted to Tae Kwon Do because it pairs quick, explosive movements with flow."

But for Panio, the playful fun begins with sparring. He compares it to dancing. "You're not intending to really hurt the person, it's all about movement and response, action and reaction. Your opponent is your dance partner. You read each other, play off each other, act as each other's shadow. It's *play* for adults. And it seems to me sometimes that the only way we can justify adult play is to disguise it in the alleged seriousness of combat."

Although it appears to be all about strategy, Tae Kwon Do is an Intuitive process. This appeals to Saffrons' need to stop the internal judgments and "get out of their heads." Panio says, "You don't have time to analyze and think. Not much time at all. You're just reacting and moving—dancing—and making tiny changes here and there. I've gone through entire workouts in the gym with free weights thinking about something else, errands, work, a book I'm reading. This has never happened in sparring. You *can't* think of anything else."

There is a spiritual element to Tae Kwon Do that also appeals to Panio. He notes that his teachers stress the fundamental spirituality of martial arts along with humility, self-awareness, cooperation, and persistence. "It's never about fighting and domination. It's always about self-mastery, about conquering fear and ego and continuing to strive for perfection, the impossible goal."

FAVORITE ACTIVITIES

Biking: This incredibly flexible activity can be intense or casual and is a great way to get outside. Saffrons want to keep their bikes handy and convenient, ready to take a spin alone or with someone who can keep up the pace. Group rides can be fun, as long as there's not too much advanced coordination involved. Saffrons with Efficiency especially enjoy the challenge of bike racing.

Cardiovascular machines and fitness classes: With their priorities of outdoor settings, convenience, and minimal process, Saffrons are unlikely to regularly use cardio machines at a fitness center unless they're part of a training program for a specific purpose. However, they might have a cardio machine at home. Saffrons with Harmony often take fitness classes if they provide the flow and music they enjoy.

Dance: With their love of movement and flow, Saffrons are drawn to dance and its opportunities for creativity. Harmonies may enjoy group classes in Salsa dancing and Jazzercise, as long as the music suits their taste and they like the way the instructor runs the class. All Saffrons respond to the creative aspect of dance.

Hiking: Hiking holds special appeal for Saffrons. It gets them outdoors and can be done at any pace. It's worth the extra couple of miles to be out beyond the urban landscape, alone or with others. Saffrons with Harmony often find a spiritual connection in nature. Saffrons with Efficiency find freedom and release in the outdoors; they might add rock climbing for an additional challenge.

Martial arts: This diverse group of traditions is appealing to Saffrons. They all involve flow and concentration in concert with intensity, controlled force, and discipline. Saffrons enjoy the philosophy behind the arts, which meshes with their own code of honor.

Roller dancing, skating, tap dancing, Ultimate Frisbee, kickball, other "fun" activities: Any physical pursuit that provides fluid movement, full body engagement, and contains an element of self-expression appeals to Saffrons.

Running: Alone, or preferably with a comfortable other, running is an activity that requires a minimal process to initiate and can be done anywhere. Running with a partner lets Saffrons share the experience and yet remain somewhat apart. Light banter with the right person is rewarding. Training for a race with others is motivating and keeps it interesting. When alone with an iPod full of favorite music, it's easier.

Walking: Another great way to get outdoors, walking offers the ease of entry and the flexibility that appeal to Saffrons. Harmonies like to see where the path takes them. Efficients enjoy letting the walk serve double duty—engaging in a physical activity with a destination in mind, or a conversation with a colleague.

Yoga: Various schools of yoga can serve as both a challenge and a pathway to spirituality for Saffrons. Studying the philosophy is an additional enticement. Saffrons will turn to yoga for the fluidity, with each posture naturally flowing into the next. They often enjoy intense yoga practices like Bikram. Yoga typically offers a way to do their own thing and still be part of a group of similarly engaged people.

ROADBLOCKS AND TIPS

Roadblocks:

- Boredom
- Ignoring physical needs and allowing other interests to trump physical activity

- Inconvenience
- Perfectionism and self-criticism

Top 10 Tips

1. Anything that seems like pure exercise is boring and difficult to sustain. Choose activities that allow you to focus on something else and get exercise along the way.

2. Take part in outdoor activities as much as possible. Saffrons find the outdoors especially appealing and energizing.

3. Identify multiple venues, for variety and spontaneity. Locate environments near home and work for easy logistics.

4. Respond to your inclination for flow. Keep your gear handy and in ready-to-go condition so you can be your spontaneous self. Optimize your chances for success by minimizing the stops and starts that interfere with flow. Go to the gym in workout clothes to avoid wasted time in the locker room.

5. If you train in a gym, shop for the right gym—one that's unfussy, where you feel like yourself and where you're able to take part as you choose and dress to be comfortable.

6. Choose activities that appeal to your fun, playful side. Those that allow for self expression are especially important to Saffrons with Harmony. Avoid structured activities with rigid attendance requirements.

7. Download your favorite music on your iPod and take it with you when walking or running. It will make all the difference and keep your energy up.

8. Take part in solitary activities alongside others. With a comfortable person, light banter can provide just the right amount of engagement to spark your energy.

9. Choose activities and environments that provide enough distraction to calm your internal critic and "get you out of your head."

10. Train for an event—a great way to beat boredom, focus your interest, feel challenged, and spend time with like-minded people. But carefully select competitive atmospheres that allow you to remain positive and satisfied. Separate exercise from competency in other areas.

SAFFRON WORDS

Challenge, convenient, flexible, flow, focus, freedom, fun, impromptu, intense, like-minded people, natural, options, play, self expression, strategy, unfussy

Saffrons at a Glance—Saffron Seeking: Making Workouts into Play

INTP: Saffron Efficiency—Dominant Introverted Thinking with Auxiliary Extraverted Intuition

INFP: Saffron Harmony—Dominant Introverted Feeling with Auxiliary Extraverted Intuition

Overall Qualities	Saffrons are attracted to activities that are flexible and convenient and provide an opportunity for spontaneity and self-expression. Anything too organized tends to fade out. Easily bored and internally demanding, Saffrons enjoy challenging activities with the right combination of fun, freedom, and flow. A sense of play is appealing, making fun activities, either alongside like-minded others or solo, a high priority.
Motivation:	• Difficult, interesting, fun challenges • Physical activities that benefit body, mind, and spirit • Reducing internal stress and boosting energy through exercise
Approach:	• Seek a combination of challenge, fun, freedom and flow in an activity that is personally appealing • Prefer minimal process and limited advanced planning • Appreciate flexibility that supports enjoyment of serendipity

Focus:	• Establish flow, create rhythm, and keep it going • Music to engage the mind and maintain flow • A goal creates focus and intensity
Environments:	• Seek natural surroundings and fresh air • Connect to nature, appreciating the freedom it provides • Prefer outdoor cardio activities, with minimal logistics • Opt for fitness center with an unfussy atmosphere, without pressure to "dress"
Interpersonal Connections:	• Solitary activities alongside comfortable others, easily coordinated • Enjoy training for an event with like-minded others • Engaged by undemanding banter with others • Choose group classes with good music and flow • Nourished by exercise alone, which can provide reflection time
Sample Quotes:	*It feels natural to be outside. I enjoy biking with others, as long as we're on the same skill level. I'm not going to bike with the wrong person more than once. I can get easily bored and only go to the gym for a specific purpose, like lifting weights. I intentionally take mental rests from time to time. It removes the pressure.* *Saffron Efficiency* *I have to distract or entertain myself in order to exercise. It's got to be fun. I can't imagine anything more dreadful than exercising in a lockstep platoon with the drill sergeant barking commands. It doesn't work to get pitted against someone else. Pleasure in the activity is a much better motivator.* *Saffron Harmony*

CHAPTER 9

INJ, The White Canvas: Trailblazers on Familiar Paths

INTJ – Dominant Introverted Intuition with Auxiliary Extraverted Thinking
INFJ – Dominant Introverted Intuition with Auxiliary Extraverted Feeling

A blank canvas stands on an easel, pure white and receptive to the inner visions of the artist's creative mind. It's the perfect representation of this inventive type, with their connection to the unconscious that yields an endless stream of ideas and visions. Whites deal in imagery and abstractions, much as the artist uses color and form, to represent what can't be put into words.

Whites are independent, guided by an internal compass rather than by any external forces. They are confident of their Intuition, trusting their own judgments and perceptions more than those of others. They just know. For Whites, something is judged to be right or wrong based on whether it supports or contradicts their inner visions or knowing.

This type is attracted to complexity. Unlike Blues who want to simplify, Whites add levels and layers to every task to fully describe the complexity of their personal vision. For example, one White with Efficiency described a highly detailed chart he created for his committee at work. He was frustrated because it wasn't complex enough to communicate his ideas. His co-workers were frustrated because it was so complex they didn't understand it.

Easily wrapped up in their ideas, Whites are happy to work alone or with a few trusted and competent colleagues. They'll share their ideas only when the moment is right. Naturally introspective, Whites receive visions rather than create them. Whites are the true trailblazers, whose thoughts and ideas are often way ahead of their time (but note that in order to let their ideas soar, they need the comfort of routine and familiarity).

Whites are intrigued by this bustling internal world. While not reclusive, they are more stimulated by their mental musings than by the outer world. As Maureen, a

White with Efficiency, surmised: "I have nothing against travel, I just feel there is so much of my own mind I haven't explored and I would rather see what's there."

With so much going on inside, Whites seek an outer world that's orderly, organized, and predictable. They seek familiar pathways that provide environmental stability as their minds soar. Chaos is disturbing, and a disorganized space is unsettling and nagging. Incomplete tasks destroy Whites' concentration. They are calmed by e-mails answered, letters mailed, reports handed in, and decisions made.

Unlike quick-moving Silvers, this type is deliberate and slower-paced. Whites' inner focus prevents them from being carried by external momentum and flow. They need time to reflect, and time to transition from one activity to the next. They don't like being rushed and are easily jarred or startled.

For Whites with their preference for Introverted Intuition, exercise and physical activity serve a particularly valuable function beyond the obvious benefits of improved health and fitness. When they are alone and their bodies are physically engaged in familiar activity, the experience becomes a kind of moving meditation. Whites can let their minds drift into a zone in which they can receive their most creative and complex ideas from the unconscious. Alyx, a White with Efficiency, describes her hikes alone in the woods as "a place of serenity and early cosmic connection." This experience, she said, would not be available to her sitting still.

MOTIVATION, APPROACH, FOCUS

Activities that allow for calming mental drift and the opportunity for reflection rank at the top of Whites' list. They find most appealing exercise that includes the hum of repetitive motion without demanding too much focus and attention. This preference is reflected in Doug's (White with Efficiency) description of running: "A good run is one

---

I prefer a bare room for yoga practice, but the one I do have works pretty well. I have some things in it, but everything is straightened out so there's nothing to grab my attention and give me an excuse not to practice.

—Meg, White with Harmony

that gives me an opportunity to reflect, but it's a very passive reflecting. It's not thinking about something; it's just kind of letting things pop up."

Whites approach exercise as they do everything else, with planning and structure, after sufficient reflection. Reflection, in fact, is a hallmark of their personality. They don't jump head first into anything, including fitness, and the lag time between having an idea and putting it into action can be considerable. Whites want a full-blown plan in place before starting.

With dominant Introverted Intuition pulling attention toward their inner life, Whites find that establishing a physically active adult life is easier if they've lived an active life in their youth. Without this background, they can bask in the comfort of their interesting inner world and neglect exercise. Mental musing can take the place of actual physical activity. Coupled with their penchant for establishing a meticulous plan before taking any action, starting a fitness program can be difficult.

A White with Harmony colleague and I discussed my research and what I was learning about exercise and its relationship to type preferences. Lee wasn't exercising and wanted to start a program. She hadn't lived a physically active life, so beginning was a challenge. We explored some possibilities. Like many Whites with Harmony, she's an avid reader, with outstanding powers of concentration. I suggested she consider a stationary bike for her home, because it only requires leg rotation, and of all the cardio machines it's the most compatible with reading. This concept was new to her and she liked the idea that she could read and get her exercise at the same time.

I posed a question: "So, Lee, what are you going to do next?"

Her response was "Read about stationary bikes." Lee was beginning a process where Whites always do, at the information-gathering stage. As radical and inventive as their thoughts may be, actions are researched and well-planned.

Much thought goes into each element of a White's exercise program—and a program it is, complete with categories for cardio, strength, and flexibility, and even classifications such as social, light, moderate, and intense. Being fiercely independent, Whites' programs must be of their own creation, and they need time to do the research, check out facilities, and imagine scenarios— all preliminary elements undertaken to create a comprehensive plan. There is nothing slap-dash about this type.

Once they've made their plan and regular physical activity is in their routine, however, it becomes a cherished part of their life and doesn't easily slip out. Providing expression of their Introverted Intuition, exercise and physical activity can serve particularly valuable mental and spiritual functions. "I have not gotten off track in the ten years I have been exercising regularly," Bill, a White with Harmony, said. "I don't allow myself, and I couldn't even think of my life without exercise. It's part of who I am and what I do. The closest I've come to being without it was once when I sprained my ankle and had to take a few days' rest, but I was back in no time."

ENVIRONMENT AND PERSONAL CONNECTIONS

Whites seek comfort and familiarity in their exercise environments. Bike paths they've been on before, orderly gyms with dumbbells neatly racked, and fellow participants who stay on task all rank high. When Whites include a gym workout in their weekly schedule, their preference is to find a place that's small and uncrowded.

Evelyn, a White with Harmony, routinely attends a Spinning class at six a.m. several days a week. "I go to the club when it is not populated and I can get in and out," she said.

Characteristically, Whites prefer keeping a low profile at the gym, and they're turned off by "seen and be seen" health clubs that one White with Harmony referred to as "meat markets."

Rudy, a White with Efficiency, chose a gym because it was off the beaten path. "I don't like to bump into people from work or other parts of my life at the gym," he said. He notices the way gym equipment is laid out and how the facility is maintained. He wonders about the logic behind the layout, but he considers amenities that aren't related to the fitness function a waste. The extras hold little appeal for Whites with Efficiency, and they're certainly not about to pay for them.

Whites with Harmony, on the other hand, are in search of a peaceful environment, and many report enjoying amenities such as well appointed locker rooms, saunas, and steam rooms.

Whites love the outdoors—hiking, camping, fishing—and enjoy completing outdoor projects. Whites with Efficiency have a rugged, individualistic personality that attracts them to the wild, even harsh, qualities of nature. If they build a lake cottage, it will likely be rustic and unadorned, fitting in with their experience of the outdoors.

Whites with Harmony have an equal appreciation of nature and enjoy outdoor projects, but their focus is on its beauty and the peaceful serenity it promises. Their cottage would be softer, finished, and lined with well-tended pots of flowering plants.

Easily jarred when reality doesn't match their vision, Whites take great pains to align the two as much as possible. Whites with Efficiency prefer spare environments. The amenities they consider "frills" are many, sometimes including elements that that the rest of the world finds appealing, such as hot running water and doors that close.

Whites with Efficiency will build a lookout positioned perfectly to catch a view of the sunset—but comfortable chairs may be considered unnecessary, and visitors might detect a small bit of criticism if they're not up to that level of rustic enjoyment.

Whites with Harmony also value a calm environment, but their idea of calm means "peaceful," rather than "rustic." Don, a White with Harmony, enjoys his living room with its beautiful view of the Green Mountains. Flowering pots line the stone patio he built himself. Outdoor chairs are placed around to provide optimum views for his family and guests. For these Extraverted Feeling types, comfortable amenities add to the peace of the environment, rather than distract from it.

Meg, a White with Harmony, describes the yoga environment she has created in her home: "The walls are painted with jewel-tone colors—green and purple. The lighting is soft. There is a water fountain and candles, and I play meditative music."

Whites with Efficiency are more inclined than Whites with Harmony to include visits to the fitness center as part of a weekly routine. Their environmental requirements are not as oriented to peace and ambience as Harmonies. However, both types prefer to keep interaction to a minimum at the

I like activity that allows me to work independently but not necessarily alone. I like to go where people are, but not be forced to interact with them every minute. For me, it's important to get away from home, from work, and treat exercise time as a little vacation from the stress of everyday life.

—Jesse, White with Harmony

gym; they're there to exercise and prefer to accomplish that with the least amount of wasted time and interruptions. Crowds and classes involving high levels of interaction aren't attractive. But a quiet yoga class might be just up their alley.

WHITES WITH EFFICIENCY (INTJ)

Whites with Efficiency are not shrinking violets. In fact, they are considered the most independent of all personality types. When they believe in something, they can be determined (some might say stubborn) and will champion their position at almost any cost. Undaunted by their detractors and unshakeable in their beliefs, they are known to pursue their vision, no matter the consequences.

This type has a strong intellectual bent and would rather deal with ideas and theories than with people and feelings. At the office, they prefer to work alone or with a few competent colleagues, polishing their ideas and not sharing them until they are ready.

This may baffle some of their more forthcoming co-workers. But Doug, a White with Efficiency, said, "I'm not trying to be secretive; it just doesn't occur to me to communicate until I'm ready."

Whites with Efficiency appreciate organization and structure; following through on their plans is calming. While they might consult fitness literature, or schedule a session or two with a trainer, they typically develop their own exercise program based on specific results they've established as important and achievable—for instance, looking better, feeling better, sleeping better, or combating stiffness. Exercise might also be a way to get in shape for other activities—weight training to increase strength for skiing, for example.

Whites with Efficiency envision and loosely plan their workouts for the week (a five-mile run on Tuesday and Thursday, thirty minutes in the weight room on Monday and Wednesday) and will stick to the schedule they create rather than respond to the outside pressures of work or family

---

Excerpt from interview with Cathy, White with Efficiency:

Q: Tell me about your yoga teachers.

A: Oh, I don't know, there's someone named Lydia, there's someone named Sandy, and I think there's a Michelle.

obligations. Unlike other types who are energized by spontaneous activities, Whites don't like being swept up in someone else's agenda and find that such activities provide no time for reflection.

Whites don't mean to be rude, but they go to a gym to work out. Chit-chat and noise are distracting, and cell phones are a special irritant to Whites with Efficiency. The operative word is quiet. To save time and avoid small talk, they visit health clubs at off-peak times, increasing the likelihood of finding fewer people in the facility. They prefer having a small number of people in the environment quietly doing similar workouts.

In addition to planned exercise indoors, designed around achieving results they've set for themselves, Whites with Efficiency love partaking in outdoor challenges. Whether it's hiking, biking, canoeing, or sailing, this type enjoys almost any activity that allows them to experience the freedom and challenge of the outdoors and be refreshed by time alone in nature with their thoughts.

An attraction to routine, with a simultaneous desire to improve, can create tension for Whites. How, for example, can you continue to get stronger by doing the same weight lifting program for years? Whites with Efficiency solve this dilemma

by creating challenges for themselves when exercising, or figuring out ways to improve and better approach their workout. At times, they may enjoy being accountable to others, as long as they've had a role in directing the activity they're participating in. This could mean biking with a group, or allowing their teenage or adult children to "set the pace" for a hike or run.

WHITES WITH HARMONY (INFJ)

Whites with Harmony are driven by insights and images of the future, much like Whites with Efficiency. Often mystical, they live with a barrage of impressions—even including premonitions about the future. But, with Feeling directed to their external world, Whites with Harmony tend to have a warm and supportive nature. Think of Glinda, the Good Witch in *The Wizard of Oz*. Like Glinda, Whites with Harmony have a protective, parental Intuition. They are good at reading people, but they don't share their awareness until they're ready.

Whites with Harmony also share an independent nature with their Efficiency partners and are no less passionate about their visions. However, a need for harmony drives their relationships, making them sensitive to and distressed by conflict. They will do what they can to prevent or avoid it.

Whites with Harmony are responsible and responsive to others, and this can weigh heavily on them. Physical activity provides a refreshing respite, giving them an opportunity to get away from it all—from work, the phone, people, requests, and family responsibilities. It's a time to de-stress, think about things, and be with their internal visions.

This type can also find it rewarding to turn off all the noise from the inner world by totally focusing on an activity. Reina, a White with Harmony and a busy financial planner in NYC, said that from time to time she enjoys exercise that demands her full attention. "For me, that's provided by dance, or dance aerobics, that has complicated choreography and patterns that force me to focus on the combinations. It's a great counter-balance to the analytical demands of my career. There's no room in my mind for anything but *right, left, right, step, turn, step*—to keep time with the music. This is a

healing respite from stress at work or in my personal life."

More than any other color type, Whites with Harmony describe their love of peaceful environments. They find large and noisy gyms especially jarring and hectic. Mear talked of her preference for being outdoors, which she described as spiritual and "my time with God."

Whites with Harmony also respond to tranquil indoor environments. For example, a simple, well appointed yoga studio with small classes appeals to their need for beauty and solitude. They typically love to garden, quietly reveling in creating pleasing spaces, feeling at peace with nature.

Whites with Harmony are most comfortable with familiar places and routines, and when trying a new activity, they look for one with an element they're already accustomed to.. They prefer working with someone known or trusted in an environment in which they have prior experience. Cameron described enrolling in a belly dancing class.

> *I use the walk as an opportunity to focus on my breath and take in the natural world around me. I allow my thoughts to move without trying to problem solve. It's a way to combine exercise with releasing the mind-chatter and connecting with something outside myself, such as nature.*
>
> —Lynn, White with Harmony

Although she'd contemplated trying it for a long time, it wasn't until her yoga teacher started the class that she moved forward. "I knew and was comfortable with her and with the fitness center where she would teach the class," Cameron said.

MEET THE WHITES

Doug, White with Efficiency (INTJ)

The entry point for Introverted Intuitive's exercise programs (and for them, there is almost always a "program" element to exercise) is often described as a *moment of occurrence*. This is a memorable moment that can be recalled years later. Doug describes his: "I've always been fit and a good athlete. I played three sports in high school and skied competitively. I enjoy hiking, biking, skiing, and the outdoors. I've always thought of myself as fit, and the necessity of a regular exercise program hadn't occurred to me until one day when I was raking leaves in the backyard.

"I was pooped and decided I didn't have the strength I ought to have. I analyzed the situation and saw there was something I could do, but many months went by before I finally started going to the gym. I tend to look at what needs to be done and approach things with deliberateness. Exercise is no different."

In White with Efficiency fashion, Doug examined the situation, decided he could do something about it, and deliberately and intentionally moved toward the goal. Eventually, he put together a fitness routine that included indoor cardio and resistance training as well as outdoor runs and bike rides. "I think ahead and work out schedules in my head," he said. "I mentally keep tabs, identify a time in which it will happen, and lock it in."

Many people experience a dilemma when they don't want to have a conversation at the gym and the individual on the next treadmill wants to chat. That is not a concern for Doug. He laughed, "I don't have a problem with that. I just don't go there and they get the message." As he says, "I go to the gym to exercise, not to do business or socialize."

Doug usually goes to his gym at noon and runs through a self-designed program of weights and cardio. Although he rarely talks to people there, he's discovered there's something stimulating about going to a place where others are doing a version of whatever he's doing.

In addition to the gym routine, he runs outdoors by himself three to four times a week, usually covering about three miles. "Running with someone else isn't fun," he said. "I like to go on my own route, gauge my stamina, and zone out when I'm running. My brain goes to another place."

He sees the benefits of exercise clearly. "Exercise strengthens me physically and mentally," he said. "It makes me feel stronger and more resilient, and it gives me energy to deal with the extraverted world. I continue to evaluate it logically. I know it makes me feel better."

Cathy, White with Efficiency (INTJ)

Cathy's approach to fitness can be summed up in three words: discipline, independence, and challenge. And in typical White with Efficiency style, Cathy creates her own structure and sets her own pace. "First thing every morning, I figure out what I am going to do for exercise," she said. "I may change my plan, but I always start with a plan."

If the weather is good, Cathy heads outdoors. Her favorite activities include kayaking, biking on country roads, or walking her dog in the woods. If she must exercise indoors to achieve her goals, she goes to a nearby fitness center, where she rides the recumbent bike as she reads work-related material.

Cathy uses a convenient gym that offers cardiovascular equipment, strength training, tennis, and yoga under one roof. She takes a variety of yoga classes and said she looks forward to them and works hard during the sessions. She particularly enjoys Astanga yoga, because in that class she breaks a sweat.

Unlike Whites with Harmony who prefer supportive yoga teachers, Cathy doesn't pay particular attention to who teaches her class. She values the teachers for their competence rather than their personal style or compatibility. When asked about her instructors, she doesn't know them by name.

Cathy describes herself as having always been competitive, with herself as well as with others. She takes pleasure in setting and achieving fitness goals. "I'm always looking for a fun challenge that makes me stretch a little to achieve it," she said. "Five years ago, I completed The Long Trail [a hiking path stretching north to south for 265 miles along the entire length of Vermont]. Four years ago, I did my first 100-mile bike trip. Right now, a friend and I are kayaking around the entire shoreline of Lake Champlain and all its major islands."

Cathy's advice to fellow Whites with Efficiency is: "Decide in the morning when you'll work out. Then, stick to your plan."

Mear, White with Harmony (INFJ)

Mear is a full time administrative assistant for a chain of quick service restaurants and a part time yoga teacher. Her route to yoga has built slowly, with each new step accompanied by a bit of the familiar.

Mear expressed an interest in Astanga yoga to a friend who gave her a DVD by Astanga yoga expert David Swenson. In the privacy of her home, Mear practiced the program for several months. When David Swenson visited her hometown to teach a week of classes, she enrolled.

"Would you have enrolled in his class without having worked out to his DVD first?" I asked.

"Heavens no!" she responded to the unthinkable. For additional familiarity, before the first class, Mear visited the yoga studio where Swenson would teach—checking out the parking, bathrooms, set-up of the room, and the general layout.

"I'm a very routine-oriented person," Mear said. "If I can figure out how to make it a routine, I will. I'm habitual."

Mear has many interests, and she plans carefully so she can incorporate them into her life. She plays the flute and recently took up rug hooking and watercolor painting. She was an active athlete growing up, partici-

pating in ice skating, gymnastics, and swimming. Quick to note that none of her fitness activities have ever been competitive, Mear said, "It's about the experience, not being judged."

Today Mear exercises most days of the week and frequently goes hiking or biking with a friend. On weekends, she prefers to be outdoors, weather permitting. "For me, including other people works best when I go to new places to hike or bike," she said. "I'm not likely to go someplace new on my own. Going with someone who's familiar with the terrain increases my comfort level with the activity."

During the week, she goes to the gym or a yoga class. "My perfect workout is doing an activity I'm comfortable with in an environment I'm accustomed to," she said. Mear packs her gym bag the night before she's going out—even packing her reading material, if the next day includes cardio at the gym.

Mear prefers to exercise alone. "At the gym, I'm very focused and do not tend to socialize," Mear said. "I'm there for a purpose. I want to get in and out in the shortest time possible."

Don, White with Harmony (INFJ)

Don is an associate director of career

services at a small, elite liberal arts college. He counsels students interested in careers in finance and regularly makes trips to New York City to call on Wall Street financial firms. His job is fast-paced, heavily inter-active, and can be hectic, depending on the time of year.

Don says he has a significant prefer-ence for exercising outside. "There are so many incredible ways to interact with the outdoors," he said. Don is passion-ately drawn to activities like biking, hiking, cross-country skiing, and gardening. He has a beautiful yard with spectacular views of the Adirondacks and enjoys designing the peaceful environment of his land-scape, taking special pleasure in the stone walls he continues to build around his property. These activities are calming, allowing for mental drift and time spent with his internal visions. As Don describes, "It's a time for my most creative internal work. I like to be in a situation where daydreams happen."

Don's engagement with outdoor activi-ties provides a time to get away from work, the phone, students, employers, and house-hold responsibilities. It's a balance to the extraverted requirements of his job.

With their reflective nature, Introverted Intuitives tend not to be quick responders. To be at their best and most comfort-able, they maximize their familiarity with their surroundings. For many years Don was a competitive biker, designing his own training program and training solo. With a White preference for knowing the terri-tory before setting out, he would arrive at races early and scope out the route. "I try to know the terrain where I will be racing. I don't do well with surprises," he said.

To supplement his solo activities, Don enjoys hiking with his wife and their young son. A short hike up a mountain when his son arrives home from school or a cross-country ski at night on a lighted trail are ideal father/son activities.

Don's physical activities outdoors match and nourish his White with Harmony spiri-tual nature. As he describes, "The woods stand for a place of quiet and natural beauty—the natural world connects us back to creation and something larger than ourselves. A place like Muir Woods [the national redwood park in California] is a living cathedral for me."

I asked his advice for other Whites with Harmony. He eloquently responded: "Find the points where your imagination and Intuition touch physical activity. Use nature as a medium."

A WHITE WITH HARMONY RETHINKS HER ENVIRONMENT

Claudia, a White with Harmony, is a former dancer in New York City. She lived overseas for many years, spending most of her time in Paris and Singapore. She'd been going to a gym to lift weights twice a week and hated every minute of it, in spite of the fact that she'd found a trainer she liked very much.

The trainer, a former dancer like Claudia, was personable and knowledgeable. The two communicated well, and Claudia felt respected and cared for. But she found it difficult to go to the gym, where the jarring atmosphere conflicted with her preference for peaceful environments.

I spoke with her about the 8 Colors of Fitness program, and how her gym choice might be clashing with her personality type. She had a flash of insight. "I will wear my ballet tights," she said. "And we can lift weights in the adjoining studio—a calmer room that has a ballet barre in it."

These adjustments transformed the weight routine. Claudia enjoys feeling like a dancer again, and the peaceful and familiar atmosphere of the studio has enabled her to enjoy weight lifting more than she ever thought possible. She actually looks forward to the sessions now.

FAVORITE ACTIVITIES

Biking: On a few favorite routes, away from busy interactions, without trucks whizzing by, the quiet of the bike wheels' rotation carries Whites to the calm space they enjoy. Alone is best, although a familiar person who can keep up works also. To prepare for a race, Whites should study the route and terrain to learn what to expect.

Cardiovascular equipment: Organize activities into categories, perhaps including a few weekly visits to the gym to put some time in on the treadmill, stepper, or stationary bike. Not inclined to spend social time at the gym, Whites should go at time when they can get in and out quickly.

Hiking: For seekers of tranquil environments, hiking is ideal. It can be made easy or more difficult by changing the terrain and speeds.

Strength Training: Most Whites, especially those with Efficiency, include strength training as part of their fitness regimen. Programs are typically self-designed through research and are organized by muscle groups. Bands, dumbbells, barbells, and/or weight machines are employed.

Tai Chi: This ancient moving meditation can be practiced alone or with others—inside or outdoors. Whites find the philosophy behind Tai Chi interesting and appreciate the mind-calming benefits.

Walking: Walking pleases Whites in many ways. It has a calming repetitive motion, can be done alone or with a few others, is performed outside in the tranquility of nature, and provides a respite from the world. And while the feet are on autopilot, active minds can drift a million miles away. Labyrinths hold special appeal.

Yoga: The body/mind/spirit connection appeals to Intuitive Whites. They especially enjoy the deep learning and practice of yoga and are likely to make it a mainstay (using other activities to supplement it), and they appreciate the deep stretching yoga encourages. Yoga classes are a way to be with others while not interacting directly, but yoga practice can also be done at home.

ROADBLOCKS AND TIPS

Roadblocks:

- Postponing starting without a full blown plan
- Unfamiliar, distracting, or jarring environments
- Disruption of routine due to change of location or other demands
- Not enough time—being rushed

Top 10 Tips

1. Shrink the plan. Just begin, even without all the pieces in place.
2. Accept unfinished workouts as better than no workouts; commit to just ten minutes, and pick up where you left off next time.
3. Use your natural inclination to organize into categories. Plan for cardio, stretch, and strength training.
4. Try before you buy. Familiarize yourself with the facility and develop comfort

with the layout before you actually go for a workout. Visit the gym at different times of operation so you can choose an un-crowded time that best provides a conducive atmosphere.

5. Carefully select environments that aren't distracting. Work out in calm and tranquil spaces that encourage relaxed exercise.

6. Schedule solitary activities that provide balance to work, family, and other responsibilities.

7. Designate time to plan ahead for fitness activity on the road; research resources and locations and make a plan. Organize routines around activities that use portable equipment, such as DVDs, resistance bands, and yoga mats.

8. Choose activities that are repetitive, enabling mental drift and providing refreshing and creative time alone.

9. Align with your penchant for the familiar by choosing activities that you can make routine and fit into the rhythms of your life.

10. Your pace and interest in reflection make you especially sensitive to time pressure. Build buffer time on both sides of an activity to avoid feeling rushed.

WHITE WORDS

Alone, categories, challenge, comfortable, confident, disciplined, familiar, habitual, independent, meditation, organized, plan, predictable, reflective, repetitious, zone

Whites at a Glance—The White Canvas: Trailblazers on Familiar Paths

INTJ: White Efficiency—Dominant Introverted Intuition with Auxiliary Extraverted Thinking

INFJ: White Harmony—Dominant Introverted Intuition with Auxiliary Extraverted Feeling

Overall Qualities	Whites are self-organized and attracted to physical activity they can structure at their own pace. Exercise provides solitary time for reflection and visioning. Jarred by interruptions and chaos, Whites require orderly environments for exercise that provide necessary calm. Outdoor environments and familiar paths and activities are appealing, allowing exercise to become a moving meditation. Advanced planning makes it happen.
Motivation:	• Calming reflection encouraging internal visions • Executing planned program • Attraction to body/mind/spirit connection • Interacting with the outdoors
Approach:	• Organize program according to own vision • Classify exercise into categories and shape program accordingly • Plan and structure in advance • Comforted by routine and repetition

Focus:	• Internal focus encourages creativity • Mind can go elsewhere • Excellent concentration allows reading while engaged in repetitious cardio activities
Environments:	• Comfortable and familiar fitness center • Tranquil, calm environment • Outdoors when possible
Interpersonal Connections:	• Prefer quiet • Small, familiar groups okay • Chit-chat is distracting
Sample Quotes:	*I prefer exercising alone. I belong to a fitness club which is "off the beaten path" so I don't run into people with whom I socialize or do business. I tend to go at off-peak times to avoid crowds. I don't like external distractions when I am exercising…like cell phones and people gossiping.* White Efficiency *The environment needs to be peaceful. Stimulation from the outer environment must be kept to a minimum if I am able to find the points where my imagination and Intuition touch physical activity. I practice yoga indoors in a meditation room with jewel tone colors—green and purple, a water fountain, candles, and soft lighting.* White Harmony

CHAPTER 10

ENJ, Royal Purple: Pursuers with a Plan

ENTJ: Dominant Extraverted Thinking with Auxiliary Introverted Intuition
ENFJ: Dominant Extraverted Feeling with Auxiliary Introverted Intuition

Friendly, outgoing, and energetic, this type walks with confidence and speaks with certainty. The royal color Purple describes them well. Purples don't seek the limelight, but are not uncomfortable with it. As Extraverts with Introverted Intuition, they can frequently be initiators of cutting-edge ideas and are good at anticipating societal trends well before they happen.

Purples are organized and productive, always working from a plan. That plan is referred to and updated regularly, but Purples ultimately stay with it until they accomplish what they set out to do. They expect a lot from themselves and from others.

With a strong sense of purpose, they express little doubt about their aims as they set out to bring their environment under control as much as possible. Purples appreciate matters unfolding without too many surprises or unexpected changes in direction.

Decision-making comes easily to Purples. In fact, it guides their personalities. But with Purples (as with all types), what you see is only half the picture. As Extraverts, Purples are energized by the outer world, frequently not giving themselves enough time alone to access their more creative side. As with Golds, without time alone the tendency is to make decisions without enough information. Purples are continually making observations and seeing connections and correlations— that is, if they give themselves the time.

Purples often find exercise to be a perfect way to get that time alone. When they're engaged in a physical activity, their minds are free to wander, and this time by themselves improves decision-making.

MOTIVATION, APPROACH, FOCUS

Purples are occupied with a constant quest for increased competency and self-improvement, and they have a strong sense of the person they think they should be. One characteristic of that person is physical fitness. Purples believe they should be sufficiently disciplined to make a place and time for exercise.

Purples organize their exercise by categories, to be certain all angles are covered. While some types might find this approach rigid or unappealing, placing exercise into categories—cardio, strength training, flexibility—helps Purples with planning.

As true of other Introverted Intuitives, Purples often remember the moment when they were first motivated to begin an exercise program—the very moment when something in life pulled them up short and said, "You're not in the shape you want to be in—or need to be in." They recognized the necessity at that moment and made the decision to take action. With Introverted Intuition at the helm, the whole process happens in a flash—a flash that Purples remember even years later. And once they form the intention, Purples don't doubt their ability to take action and be effective.

Many Purples with established routines have commented that it's easier for them to exercise than not to exercise. Oriented toward getting their workout, as Extraverts they'll readily use a variety of gyms, fitness centers, and spas when they're on the road, as long as the facilities offer the needed resources. They have a greater flexibility than other types about walking into unfamiliar gyms, and they'd feel the void if they skipped exercise when away from home. Active Purples frequently report they can't remember going for more than three days without a workout.

Purples and Golds are action-oriented, Extraverted Judging types. After an information-gathering period, they each like to make a decision and get going. But the two diverge in their Perceiving function—Introverted Intuition for Purple, Introverted Sensing for Gold. So, while Golds believe in *a right way* established by professionals or credentialed authorities, Intuiting Purples are confident

I'm a strong strategic thinker and I like to deal with people from strength. Exercise helps that. I mentally perform better when exercise is part of my day.

—Karen, Purple with Efficiency

they can devise the best way for themselves. Purples will research, study, consult authorities, and do whatever is needed to collect information. However, with confidence and independence as trademarks of this color type, they trust their own ability to pull together a plan.

Purples may sporadically participate in competitions, including walkathons, marathons, and bike races, and they enjoy the variety of activities that accompany training for an event. Similarly, they may like to experiment occasionally with novel fitness approaches, just to liven things up. Variety adds spice, but eventually, Purples return to what they can make routine.

As Introverted Intuitives, Purples enjoy the chance to "zone out" and, once engaged, don't need to be pushed while exercising. Their motivation is internal. Kathryn, a Purple with Harmony and professional road bike racer, described her reaction to crowds near the end of a race who call out, "You're almost there."

"It definitely doesn't encourage me," she said. "It distracts me. I'm in a zone where I don't worry about the finish line. I know what's going on in my head and I know what it takes to finish. I have a lot of internal monologue that works for me. When people inter-rupt my internal monologue, it doesn't help."

The occasions when Purples zone out during exercise can be among the most creative for them. When they work out alone, they can access their Introverted Intuition, which opens up new ideas. Take Karen, for example. She's the CEO of a communications company who explained why she likes biking: "I can get on my bike with a problem and come up with a solution. Not long ago, I got on my bike knowing I had a talk about leadership coming up. When I got off my bike an hour later, the whole presentation was structured in my mind."

Once exercise takes on an established pattern, Purples comfortably maintain a routine. They'll easily accept the need to pack their bag, and they calmly follow standard locker room procedures. Unlike Silvers and Saffrons, for whom the importance of minimizing process rises to the top, ritualized routines are okay with Purples. It doesn't feel like a waste of time if they've planned for it.

Though attitudes about and overall tendencies for approaching activity converge for all Purples, end goals for this color strongly diverge between the Thinking and Feeling dimensions that characterize

Efficiency and Harmony. Purples with Efficiency seek competence—they want to be at the top of their game. Purples with Harmony want to be better people—life is a journey toward improvement. Exercise fits nicely into each of these goals.

ENVIRONMENT AND PERSONAL CONNECTIONS

Purples' ability to sustain an exercise program is dependent on their success with maintaining control over their environment. With their Perceiving function as Introverted Intuition, for example, they're easily jarred when the physical setting doesn't suit their taste or design. Nan is a good example of this trait; when other members of her gym steered the environment in a direction she didn't enjoy, she dropped her membership.

Because Purples view exercise as a means to fitness, spending time with others is not the point. Purples care greatly about where they get their exercise. For them, the fitness center or gym is a "work environment." They want functionality, logical organization, orderly and clean facilities, and a sense of positive energy. You won't find a Purple in a gym without these qualities for long.

Purples are energized by the presence of others in their exercise environment—but *not* necessarily by interaction with them. They aren't spurred on by keeping a conversation going with a fellow runner during a race, for example. Conversation takes them out of their zone, which, after all, is a prime source of their energy.

This preference became evident mid-way through the research for this book, when I began to perceive the way exercises patterns related to type. A personal incident made this aspect of my own Purple with Harmony type clear to me.

I was running a 5K race with hundreds of others. As we were settling into our paces, a friend pulled up beside me and started to

> *Efficiency is important. I want to do as much as I can in as short a time as possible. If I employed a trainer, the purpose would be to increase my efficiency. The trainer would adjust weights, gauge which muscles need to be used, help me sculpt my body, keep track of everything*
>
> —Alexia, Purple with Efficiency

chat, something that she was quite comfort-able doing as a Saffron with Efficiency. I was jarred by the pull to be in a conversa-tion, and I knew that I would lose my energy and focus if we talked. I felt rude but knew immediately this was a situation I wanted to avoid. I said to my friend with a blunt-ness that surprised me, "Margy, I don't talk in races." Happily and with energy, I created my own space so I could get in the zone, enjoy the race, and run well.

Working from a loosely envisioned plan, Purples will typically go to the gym several days a week on their own, establishing comfort and continuity through routine. Too much scheduling and coordination with others wouldn't serve this preference. In fact, accommodating someone else's clock could cause a Purple to miss an exercise opportu-nity. Exercise falls into the job category, and organizing it around a personal relation-ship can be counterproductive and quite stressful.

Purple women's choices are frequently luxurious. I interviewed a hardworking Purple with Efficiency marketing executive, Liz, who lives in London. She described spending "a disproportionate amount" of her income on a lavish hotel spa and fitness center. Her favorite thing in the world was to complete a great workout on the tread-mill or elliptical machines, followed by reading *The Economist* in the sauna. She'd spend half a day at this regimen. Liz tried inviting friends along, but she realized the spa was best enjoyed privately, so she stopped giving invitations in order to savor this pleasure by herself.

PURPLES WITH EFFICIENCY (ENTJ)

Decisive, logical, and persistent, Purples with Efficiency believe that hard work is the most necessary ingredient of achieve-ment. With their hands on the wheel, they're always moving forward, progressing toward their goals, and aiming to be their best. Decisive and hard-driving, these natural leaders benefit from time alone during exercise to engage their auxiliary function of Introverted Intuition. It gives them an opportunity to take in more infor-mation and access the bigger picture. They frequently gravitate toward repetitious exercise in the gym or the outdoors, estab-lishing comfort with a routine that doesn't require focused attention.

Purples with Efficiency are easily recog-nized by their erect posture and stately bearing. They like winning the mental edge that comes with competence, and the environments they choose for exercise are logically structured to support this goal.

Purples don't make excuses for themselves and are impatient with excuses from others, sometimes to the point of being blunt. No one wants to look foolish, but for Purples with Efficiency the projection of competency is critical. As we'll see when we meet Nan, a Purple with Efficiency, her successful approach to exercise includes avoiding environments where she's at a disadvantage and unable to perform up to her standards.

PURPLES WITH HARMONY (ENFJ)

Vivacious Purples with Harmony take a positive, enthusiastic view of life. Realizing human potential—their own and that of others—is a driving force for them. Promoting an external world of harmony, good will, and friendly relationships provides a context for their personal approach to life. Confident and decisive, they want to go as far as they can to influence and manage their family-and-friends network. They encourage all to "be what we can be."

As Extraverted Judging types, Purples with Harmony naturally accept, and are grounded in the stability of, societal standards. At the same time, they enjoy putting their mark on things and applying a creative spin to their mode of dress, to activities and events, and even to commonly held ideas or theories.

Psychologically oriented and informed by Introverted Intuition, they (like Whites with Harmony) are fascinated by visions and perceived connections that help them to understand complex situations and interactions. However, unlike Whites with Harmony who prefer Introversion and tend to keep these insights to themselves until just the right moment, Purples with Harmony are Extraverts who readily share their understanding of situations to help others.

Comfortable with routine, Purples with Harmony pursue physical exercise in the organized fashion typical of their type. All it takes is a bit of intention with some planning and follow-through to bring regular activity into the mix. Like Purples with Efficiency, they feel like something is missing if exercise falls away.

Purples with Harmony choose friendly and orderly environments to support their goals, with a minimum of discord or distraction. Typically, they don't look for much social interaction while they exercise. They are successful when they avoid exercise environments where their attention is drawn away from their workout by personal interactions. (However, some Purples with Harmony report success with scheduled walks with a walking buddy.) With their attention so often on other people and on maintaining relationships, Purples with Harmony find peace by dropping out and withdrawing for a time. They even say they avoid engaging a personal trainer, as the sessions can become hopelessly personal, losing sight of their fitness goals.

Repetitious activity and familiar routines help Purples with Harmony relax and retreat to their inner world. Activities such as biking, running, swimming, and walking—even following a weight lifting routine while watching CNN—can be appealing.

MEET THE PURPLES

Dick, Purple with Efficiency (ENTJ)

Dick is a physician and a pilot who holds the rank of general in the National Guard. Now retired from medicine, he and his wife divide their time between a house on Cape Cod and an apartment in Florida. At age sixty-three, Dick has not lost his military bearing. Tall and fit, he walks and moves with confidence, always seeming to know exactly where he's going.

"I'm disciplined about life and disciplined about exercise," Dick said, showing his true Purple nature.

Purposeful exercise entered Dick's life more than forty years ago—a moment he remembers well—when he read a report of injuries suffered by pilots who were not in top physical condition. Ensuring that he remained in shape to fly became a goal. True to his Purple type, Dick set about creating a plan for himself, first gathering information from a broad cross-section of sources.

"I studied exercise recommendations and routines from NASA, IBM, and the NFL," he recalls. "I wanted a program that would provide maximum efficiency."

Dick's experience is typical. As stated earlier, Introverted Intuitive types frequently report knowing the moment when they decided to begin exercising. "I started because I didn't want to lose control of that plane," Dick said. "Now I just feel better doing it."

With typical Purple planning—complete

with categories—Dick describes his routines. "I swim every day, do weights three times a week, and play tennis three to four times a week," he said. "When I travel, I always book a hotel with a gym. I can't remember the last time I went seventy-two hours without exercising."

Dick's weight-lifting routine is a series of targeted workouts. "There are eight to ten muscle groups, and I organize my workouts around them," he said. He is impatient with wasted effort. "I've designed my programs for maximum efficiency. The only thing you have to sell in life is time. I don't babble with people on the phone and don't open funny attachments on e-mails."

Dick's highly accomplished life reflects an intention to live at the top of his game—the way so many Purples with Efficiency describe their motivation. During our interview, my curiosity was piqued. "How important is competition in exercise?" I asked.

Dick shot back, "Exercise is *not* a competitive sport. I exercise to stay in shape."

Nan, Purple with Efficiency (ENTJ)

Like Dick, Nan designs her workouts according to various categories and has easily integrated exercise into her life. Proud of her appearance and willing to invest effort to maintain it, Nan exercises three to four days a week, incorporating a great deal of variety in her program to provide interest. During our interview, she spoke decisively and directly, describing her likes and dislikes for physical activity, exhibiting a strong sense of having her act together, following a plan, and remaining on top of things.

Nan is an attractive woman who has owned a fashionable woman's clothing business for more than twenty-five years, during which she has effectively responded to and overcome competition and changes in this challenging industry. Nan is always well dressed, with accessories that contribute to a "total" look. Women often turn to her for advice on how to "put themselves together," home territory for a Purple.

[ENTJs] are excellent at establishing order, whether on paper, in their everyday lives, or at a business meeting. With a good sense of facts, they bring clarity into emotional situations. They are assets on any committee; they know Robert's Rules of Order and when to apply them.
—Daryl Sharp, *Personality Types: Jung's Model of Typology* (1980)

Nan said she enjoys exercising outdoors, weather permitting—no small consideration in the northeastern states. She particularly enjoys hiking, biking, in-line skating, skiing, and walking, providing options for all the seasons of the year in the mountainous area where she lives.

True to type, Nan has organized her exercises by category. For strength training, she works out on a Bowflex machine at home in her basement. In addition, she takes a Pilates class once a week at a downtown studio, which she describes as "a beautiful space and immaculately clean." Her Purple preference for manageable routines and an orderly environment is evident.

She mentioned that Weight Watchers® created activity classifications for light, moderate, or heavy exercise, and Nan applied the concept to her own life. She decided that she'd put housework down as light activity, and she now embraces it under that category. Walking with a friend is in the moderate column of general physical activities to sustain overall fitness.

Nan's choice of Pilates, on other hand, is based primarily on going after results. "It's really good, gets you a really strong stomach," she said. "I do stuff I don't want to do for the results. However, there's one thing I do love, and that's ballet," she added. "If I had time, I would take a ballet class every day." She enjoys it for the precision and discipline, as well as for the competence.

Her Purple preference for maintaining a level of control over the environment also came across during our conversation. Nan had belonged to a fitness center, but had recently let the membership lapse. "I now hate going to the gym," she said. "The younger, buff guys were treating me like a middle-aged woman. They played music I didn't like. The TV was always tuned to sports channels. I had no control over what was happening there." This is not a set of circumstances a Purple would tolerate for long. Instead, Nan devised alternate means to achieve her fitness goals and left the uncomfortable environment behind.

"As a kid, I didn't play sports because I wasn't a very good runner," Nan recalled. "However, I was a cheerleader. Whatever I yelled, the people in the stadium yelled back the same thing. I loved that." Nan fondly remembers this opportunity to lead others.

When I asked what types of exercise turn her off, she was quick to respond: "I hate running. I never snowboard. Extreme stuff doesn't appeal to me. I hate all the kid stuff and I avoid games and competition. I don't want to look stupid."

Ada, Purple with Harmony (ENFJ)

Ada was a popular career counselor and pre-law advisor at a large university for ten years. She's slim with long legs and moves gracefully and confidently in the world, naturally connecting with people and using affectionate names for others.

True to type, Ada thinks of exercise in categories. But in addition to common classifications like cardiovascular, strength training, and flexibility, Ada sees her fitness activities woven into the broader fabric of her life, involving mental, emotional, and spiritual categories, as well.

"It's about being the best we can be on every level: compassionate, intellectual, spiritual, and physical," she said. "I wouldn't want to be the kind of person who doesn't exercise, who doesn't take care and doesn't appreciate her body. There are things I use as a compass in my life," she said. "I wonder who is the fullest person I can be."

Ada's mainstay activity is yoga, and she attends one class a week with her teacher, Jennifer, whom she "loves." She talked about her search for the right teacher and the right environment: "I wanted to avoid the yoga rock stars in town whose classes have gotten too crowded," she said. "I've actually gotten to a class but turned around and gone home when I saw the rows of shoes lined up outside. I've stopped going to yoga studios because they were not clean or kept up," she said. "Places need to be important to the people who are running them—like they're hosts and it's a sacred space." Overfilled, unkempt classrooms didn't resonate with Ada's preference for attending to her spirit along with maintaining fitness.

Purples with Harmony tend to develop personal relationships with teachers and trainers, and Ada has done this with Jennifer, but she turns to her own judgment and her own resources to shape an overall program. "I go to one class a week for Jennifer to correct my technique," Ada said, "but I really enjoy doing the postures by myself. At home, I practice yoga in a beautiful little guest room overlooking our large yard. The room has yellow walls with southern exposure. It's very peaceful, serene, and bright. It's a sacred space."

Though she appreciates variety in exercise from time to time, including walking and free weights, Ada also finds familiarity attractive. "I have an affinity toward the word *routine*, but the word *rhythm* fits better," she said. Rhythm and routine allow her mind to wander during an activity. Practicing yoga postures at home or following a rhythmic free weight program at her own pace work well.

Ada enjoys the proximity of others in her class, even though she's really maintaining a sense of her private environment in the midst of the group. As a dominant Extraverted Feeling type, she fulfills a desire for connection, at the same time making room for her auxiliary Introverted Intuition. "I'm in my own private space once the class starts," she said. "It's nice to have others across the room but not interacting; I'm glad they're there. I need a lot of alone time *and* a lot of connecting."

Another situation exemplifies Purples' need that exercise be free from distracting interactions. "I walk to work several days a week for exercise," Ada said. "I always pass a friend's house and, knowing that, he asked me to stop in. Well, I can't do that. I could never be present and that bothers me—not being present." The walk to work, all the way to work, was an opportunity to exercise; Ada wanted to complete the task, not stop for a social visit. Trying to be with her friend socially while her mind was on finishing her walk would cause tension and leave her dissatisfied with both experiences. Ada considered it best to avoid mixing the two. If she'd chosen to get her exercise by walking to a friend's home for a visit, the task and the social aspect would no longer be in conflict—changing the context would make all the difference.

Entwined in Purples' desire to complete a task is their interest in self-improvement. "I think always about *depth,* which combines competence with pushing my limits," Ada said. "Doing something I never thought I could is part of depth. I push myself to the next higher limit." For Purples with Harmony, life is a journey to a better self— physically, spiritually, and in every other way.

Wyatt, Purple with Harmony (ENFJ)

Wyatt goes to the gym at five a.m. four days a week. At that time, he usually sees the same faces, and he enjoys the familiarity. He doesn't have to keep a steady conversation going, but gym members exchange casual bits of news and pleasantries, providing just enough contact.

Wyatt follows a consistent routine that includes a twelve-minute treadmill warm-up and various programs in weight training focused on specific muscle groups.

It doesn't occur to him to leave out the parts he doesn't like.

"I hate working my legs," he said. "The mornings I know I have to do legs, I need an attitude adjustment." He knows all the elements of his routine are important and he does them all. This is a matter of values, and covering all bases is part of the goal. Exercising regularly reflects how much Wyatt believes in taking care of himself.

Establishing a consistent pattern helps him sustain the momentum. His exercises are organized into a routine that he can follow even with other people around him. "I feel healthier and happier because I exercise," Wyatt said. "I can get over-focused on caring about other people, and exercise gives me permission to pay attention to myself."

A former clergyman, Wyatt retired to Maine, where he tends an apple orchard on his land. In addition to weight training at the gym, he runs regularly, and on weekends he works in the orchard and keeps busy gardening—both activities that also fall into the category of exercise.   .

On the days he runs, Wyatt prefers to be outdoors. "It's wonderful alone time," he said. "It keeps me connected to some-

thing I've been doing for a long time, so I don't slack off. I like the results."

Wyatt said he started running in 1971, doing three miles a day, six days a week. He kept up that regimen until, when he was about forty-eight years old, he hurt his knee and had to stop running to let it heal. That was when he started doing weights. Now he follows an established weekly schedule, including the weekend gardening and orchard work.

"My brain works better and clearer, and exercise gives me a sense of accomplishment," Wyatt said. "I push through it." He said he sees a connection between following through on his physical routine and his mental health and his ability to cope with emotional issues overall. "I can get through them, too," he said.

As a boy, Wyatt played sports like football and soccer in school, but he struggled with his weight, and he's careful not to let it get out of hand again. He said the gym routines help him keep his weight in check. "Both of my brothers had heart difficulty," he said. "I think about my heart."

He started doing gym workouts using a trainer to show him proper technique, something he said he doesn't do in a "natural, flowy way" on his own. "Primarily, the trainer kept me honest," he said. "He was encouraging and knowledgeable. He was young, good, and effective. We developed a wonderful relationship."

Wyatt said he'd advise other Purples with Harmony to look at exercise as an important aspect of their life and give themselves permission to pay attention to themselves by including physical activity in their schedules. "The issue is how much you care about yourself."

FAVORITE ACTIVITIES

Biking: Purples use bike riding as one component in their cardiovascular mix. As with running, others may be present, but there is no need to interact. If Purples train for a biking event, it will typically be by themselves, with occasional group sessions for variety.

Cardiovascular machines: As long as they get the cardio they're after, Purples don't mind the form it takes. They will readily use treadmills, StairMasters, elliptical machines, a stationary bike. Once their program is set, Purples enjoy seeing a few people in the gym for a boost of energy.

Pilates: Purples with Efficiency can frequently be found in Pilates studios, attracted to the organization, structure, and targeted results they get from the workouts. Pilates is great for posture, an important consideration for Purples with Efficiency.

Running: Though running is usually a solitary pursuit, Purples may join a group or a few other runners for occasional variety, for training sessions, or on special occasions, but the company of others is not the motivation.

Strength Training: Purples organize weight routines that hit each muscle group. Once they have the routines down, light distraction, such as television news, makes the time more enjoyable.

Swimming: Purples enjoy the sense of accomplishment they get from swimming laps. They will keep track with a clock or count laps to measure their progress and know when they have completed their workout.

Walking: Another option that offers variety and flexibility, walking has many different styles to choose from—leisurely walks or aerobic walks, thinking walks or talking walks. It all depends on the mood, on the desired goal, and on how the walk fits into a routine for the week.

Yoga: The body/mind/spirit aspect of yoga appeals to Intuitive Purples. A group yoga class provides a way to be with others while not directly interacting with them. In addition, yoga can be easily practiced home alone, with music or a DVD. The stretching benefits of yoga fits nicely into the flexibility category.

ROADBLOCKS AND TIPS

Roadblocks:

- Trying to proceed without a plan
- Exercise not integrated into lifestyle
- Undervaluing the importance of controlling the environment
- Distracted by elements of socialization

Top 10 Tips

1. Consult with a trainer or the exercise literature to design a program for initial set-up and knowledge; develop your own routine from there.

2. Identify your independent reason to exercise. Perhaps there was a moment of occurrence when you decided that "something needs to be done."

3. Envision, plan ahead, and schedule. You don't have to stick to your plan, but it's difficult to move forward without one.

4. Organize exercise into categories; e.g, cardio, strength, flexibility; light, moderate, and intense; indoor and outdoor.

5. Maintain interest by ensuring variety within a routine, and rotate throughout the week—sometimes walk with a friend.

6. Incorporate repetitious forms of exercise that do not require focused attention, allowing for automatic pilot.

7. Choose an environment that is pleasing and conducive to physical exercise. Environments that feel unpleasant can jar you out of your workout. The extra amenities a fitness center offers can make or break your workout.

8. Avoid being distracted by socialization during exercise. Purples tend to enjoy people in the environment, but not interacting directly with them. Save the interaction for later.

9. Avoid exercise that requires navigational

skills. Without comfortable landmarks, Purples can get easily lost, which creates anxiety and interferes with exercise.

10. Frame routine exercise as important alone/creative time.

PURPLE WORDS

Categories, control, disciplined, envision, hard-driving, independent, intentional, orderly, organized, plan, predictable, repetitious, rhythm, routine, variety

Purples at a Glance—Royal Purple: Pursuers with a Plan

ENTJ: Purple Efficiency—Dominant Extraverted Thinking with Auxiliary Introverted Intuition

ENFJ: Purple Harmony—Dominant Extraverted Feeling with Auxiliary Introverted Intuition

Overall Qualities	Disciplined initiators, Purples approach exercise with purpose and an objective, and always with a plan. Purples organize exercise into categories, e.g., cardio, weights, and strength. They are attracted to variety, and they experiment with different approaches from time to time, but are soon drawn back to exercise they can make routine. Purples have a consistent approach to exercise. Once it's in their life, they generally stay with it.
Motivation:	• Increased competency and self-improvement • Belief that it's important to be in shape and take care of yourself • Exercise providing balance to their lives
Approach:	• Plan training around self-defined goals, with specific purpose and objective • Seek others as a resource for information, then prefer being on their own • Classify activities into categories • Prefer routine repetitious exercise • Value body/mind/spirit connection

Focus:	• Solitary activity provides internal focus and access to their creative side • Enjoy repetitive motion, to "get in the zone" • Light news programs on TV when doing routine activities
Environments:	• Fitness center, a functional, orderly, and positive environment • Will enjoy and make use of amenities a facility offers • Outdoors is part of variety
Interpersonal Connections:	• Energized by people in facility, but not by directly interacting • Too much interaction with others requires energy and takes them out of the zone • Mixing in activities with others provides variety • Might go to gym with others—then separate to work out
Sample Quotes:	*I hike, bike, skate, ski, and walk. I also work out on a Bowflex machine and take a Pilates class once a week. I do it for the end result. I no longer go to the gym. The TV was always on sports channels, and they played music I didn't like. I had no control over what was happening.* Purple Efficiency *I like to enjoy life and feel good about myself, which includes being in shape. I loosely envision and structure my week ahead of time. I don't like it when others tell me what to do. I run, walk, bike, and use the elliptical machine at the gym. I love to be with my internal monolog.* Purple Harmony

SECTION THREE

For Professionals

CHAPTER 11

Coaches and Trainers: Working with the Colors

As a fitness professional, you know that one size does not fit all. Some clients respond well to weight-lifting regimens while others prefer outdoor activities. Some are traditional and conservative in their approach and some need variety with cutting-edge information. Some enjoy quiet solitude and others prefer a fast-paced class with energetic music.

You probably figure out these preferences over the course of a few session. But even the most thorough assessments can be hit-or-miss when it comes to determining what will really work for your client. The 8 Colors of Fitness program provides you with a shortcut, a state-of-the-art insight into who you're working with. With this information, you'll be ready to best meet your clients' needs and increase their likelihood for success. As their fitness level improves, you'll enjoy the satisfaction of watching their progress.

To use this information most effectively, begin by verifying your clients' color-coded exercise personality. Then read their chapter and review their chart. Learn the specific motivations, environments, and approaches they appreciate and expect. Now, read about and learn the top ten coaching tips for each of the colors, and discover how you can be more effective in helping your clients sustain an exercise program they'll never quit!

TOP TEN TIPS FOR COACHING BLUES

1. Safety concerns need to be recognized and addressed at the beginning. In all training sessions, Blues need to be reassured that the exercise/approach is safe and will, in fact, prevent injury. For example, emphasize the importance of stretching to avoid injury.

2. Blues have specific goals in mind when working with a trainer, and they want to chart and record them. Clarify goals and determine how progress will be measured (computer entries, cards, etc.) at the outset.

3. Blues respect authoritative research. Communicate your credentials and training experience. References to literature on exercise physiology are appreciated and add credibility to the importance of exercise.

4. Blues want an organized approach, and a well-formulated plan. They do not expect the coaching sessions to be fun.

5. Break training sessions into steps, making sure they completely understand and can master each step before going to the next. For example, demonstrate and explain in detail the muscle group being worked. Emphasize correct form and technique.

6. Once a program is developed, Blues are comfortable with routine. Make any changes incremental in progression.

7. Focus on the concrete. Don't expect Blues to improvise. Blues do not naturally trust body/mind/spirit messages from trainers.

8. In a series of training sessions, a trainer should begin with a brief review of the last session to ensure that information is secured in their minds. Blues might be silent about what they don't understand. Do not equate silence with understanding or agreement

9. Conduct sessions in private or less central area(s) of the gym to remove distractions and create privacy.

10. If possible, each training session should be held in the same space in the gym, using exactly the same equipment for each session.

Keep in Mind:

Blues with Efficiency have a pragmatic approach to fitness sessions, and want to get down to business right away.

Blues with Harmony look for a friendly, personal trainer and like to exchange pleasantries.

TOP TEN TIPS FOR COACHING GOLDS

1. Clarify the purpose for exercise. Concrete, ongoing benefits should be stressed, such as feeling better and looking better, or increased mobility. Emphasis on safe conditioning for sports is effective.

2. Agree on specific measurable goals, accompanied by a detailed plan of how you will mark progress.

3. Break down goals into manageable pieces, which meshes with Gold's systematic approach to any project.

4. Golds are concerned about safety, injury, and not over-doing. Provide the necessary reassurance of these factors, while keeping them challenged.

5. To provide extra confidence and increase compliance, communicate your credentials and training experience. Emphasize that there's a right way and wrong way to train, and you are going to teach them the right way.

6. Cite role models to inspire them—people they can identify with in terms of age, condition, and goals.

7. Show respect for the traditional approach favored by Gold. Don't suggest exercises or programs that have not stood the test of time.

8. Golds enjoy public recognition, and will respond well to displays of their achievements (pictures, certificates, ribbon, medals, member of the month, etc.). Encourage them to also reward themselves as they reach milestones.

9. Utilize their attraction to routine, planning, and thriftiness. Schedule six sessions in a row at the same time. Offer a discount on multiple sessions.

10. Create a plan to deal with disruption of routine. Golds who travel need to know how to continue their fitness regimens on the road, dealing with new gyms, new terrain, and other out of the ordinary conditions.

Keep in Mind:

Golds with Efficiency want a concrete progress report. Emphasize their accomplishments and the goals they are achieving.

Golds with Harmony enjoy positive affirmation, so preface corrections with praise. Recognize and provide for their need for personal connection, but limit it. It can easily divert the session.

TOP TEN TIPS FOR COACHING REDS

1. Create coaching sessions that are high-energy, action-oriented, fast-paced, and fun.

2. Reds need a concrete goal, preferring to train for a specific event or activity. They find it boring to simply "stay in shape." (In speaking to a Red, substitute the word training for exercise.)

3. Reds grasp information best in small doses—bulleted lists are effective.

4. Provide information that is specific and directive rather than theoretical.

5. Give immediate and continuous feedback about what's being done right (and wrong). Reds like to make corrections in the moment.

6. Incentives motivate Reds. Intermediate goals, such as small competitions, recognition, awards, and rewards work well.

A favorite treat after a workout (even during a workout) is appreciated by this type.

7. Consider pairing Red clients with others at the same level for personal training. Fun competitions will be appreciated.

8. Surprise them with variety. A mix of activities and locations is appreciated. Weather permitting, suggest moving the training session outdoors.

9. Introduce Reds to other people at the gym who are training in similar ways or have goals in common. Encourage a connection.

10. Reds easily socialize around physical activities. Put them high on your list to notify about special events and fun activities going on at the fitness center. Encourage them to bring along their friends.

Keep in Mind:

Reds with Efficiency enjoy trainers who encourage and prepare them for friendly competition with others, and for winning.

Reds with Harmony appreciate supportive trainers who exhibit caring and encourage friendly camaraderie and enjoyable competition with others.

TOP TEN TIPS FOR COACHING GREENS

1. Greens are unlikely to engage a trainer without first having a clear-cut objective, such as preparing for an outdoor challenge that is important to them.

2. Create a formatted, practical plan. Don't include anything extraneous that doesn't contribute to their goal.

3. Hold them accountable—that's why they hired you.

4. Assume that Greens will be training by themselves. Provide all information for self-sufficiency and preparedness.

5. Training outside is a favorite option. For example, you and your Green clients might run up hills with weighted backpacks in preparation for a climb they are training for.

6. Think outside the box. Greens will stay with a trainer longer if he/she can continually come up with new, preferably outdoor, activities that are fun, aligned with their goals.

7. Don't talk too much.

8. Greens are not naturally comfortable in gyms or locker rooms. Encourage them to come dressed to train, and keep the emphasis off the gym's amenities.

9. Respect their need for privacy. Don't try to connect them with other members or pressure them to attend group events.

10. Provide additional information related to the outdoor challenges they are training for. For example, physiological changes under different altitudes, or simple gear recommendations.

Keep in Mind:

Greens with Efficiency are minimalists and analytical. They enjoy a challenge and being held to a high standard by their trainer.

Greens with Harmony look for a trainer who provides the structure they don't provide for themselves. That person must align with their personal values.

TOP TEN TIPS FOR COACHING SILVERS

1. Trainers provide an incentive for Silvers to show up. Don't keep Silvers waiting. You could be giving them a reason to find something more interesting to do.

2. Start with the big picture—an overview of how the body and mind benefit from physical activity. With their attraction to complexity and natural curiosity, Silvers wants to learn about exercise science, including new findings in physiology and neurology.

3. Make sessions interesting, enjoyable, and fast paced. Although Silvers are serious about accomplishing their goals, they want the sessions to go by quickly.

4. Talking will not distract Silvers. As long as you're making sense, they enjoy the banter and it helps keep their mind off the exercise.

5. Disguise exercise in the context of experiencing something new. Mix in cutting-edge activities and information.

6. Advise Silvers against excessive monitoring, stops and starts. All this interferes with flow, which is fundamental to fast-paced Silvers. Silvers like to keep moving and don't like to pack. Let them know they can arrive at and leave the gym in their workout clothes.

7. Silvers naturally connect information. They will readily see body/mind/spirit-connections and be attracted to activities in which they can make such connections. Include this aspect in communication and recommendations.

8. Silvers enjoy activities with additional layers of association. Encourage their engagement in activities in which they are exploring, planning, connecting with others or learning something new.

9. Feedback leads to improvement, and won't be taken personally (in fact, Silvers take constructive criticism very well).

10. In a training session, start with activities that are fun, easy, and most enjoyable. Once Silvers begin, the momentum keeps them going. Starting is often the biggest obstacle.

Keep in Mind:

Silvers with Efficiency seek a professional relationship primarily for the results. They expect a trainer to be competent and respond to difficult questions.

Silvers with Harmony look for fun, personal interaction with their trainers, and for someone they enjoy spending time with.

TOP TEN TIPS FOR COACHING SAFFRONS

1. Saffrons make little use of coaches and trainers on a regular basis. They consult experts for a specific purpose, such as improving their skills in a particular sport or activity.

2. Communicate clearly the value you are adding to a Saffron's workout. For some types, your presence is enough, but not for this one. If you do not meet their needs, they will disappear. This type is unlikely to fill out survey forms or provide feedback to clubs.

3. Don't impose your own goals on Saffrons. Take the necessary time to understand their goals and develop a plan together to address these goals.

4. Saffrons are internally demanding, and enjoy a challenge. Check out with them that the sessions are appropriate to the level of challenge they are looking for. Keep sessions interesting and varied as Saffrons get bored easily

5. Saffrons are perfectionists, but also playful and fun-loving. Be attuned to which side of Saffrons' nature you're facing. On the playful side, they might like to share a training session with a partner or friend.

6. Don't try to impress a Saffron with your professional credentials. Your professional credentials mean nothing if a Saffron doesn't see you as competent.

7. With their Intuitive nature, Saffrons easily see the body/mind/spirit connections. Include this aspect in your communication and recommendations of indoor and outdoor activities.

8. Convenience and spontaneity are important. Provide assistance as to how Saffrons can effectively integrate exercise into their weekly routine.

9. With goals in mind, come up with playful surprises such as jumping rope or a running treasure hunt. They want to have fun but don't want to waste time.

10 Saffrons are disinclined to take the time to change clothes in the locker room or use facility amenities on a regular basis. Encourage clients to come dressed to begin the workout immediately.

Keep in Mind:

Saffrons with Efficiency will work with a trainer to learn specific skills or improve performance.

Saffrons with Harmony want to partner with trainers who understand their values. They won't tolerate experiencing their values being invalidated.

TOP TEN TIPS FOR COACHING WHITES

1. Whites have a high need to feel comfortable in a fitness facility. Give them a thorough tour of facility. Show them the equipment and various spaces to build familiarity.

2. Whites tend to set up their own fitness programs, after study and reflection. If they do consult a trainer, they're looking for specific information. Trainers should communicate that they respect White's independent approach.

3. When describing training principles and objectives, begin with an overview before going into details. The overview should address exercise in categories (flexibility, strength, cardio).

4. The only way Whites can use information is when they can organize it. Present it systematically, with no random tips, lessons, or suggestions. Stay with the plan. Whites don't appreciate surprises.

5. Give them time; this type does not like to be rushed. Don't pack too much into a session, but leave time for reflection.

6. With their Intuitive nature, Whites readily see the body/mind/spirit connection. Explore this aspect in your communication and recommendations of indoor and outdoor activities.

7. Training sessions are viewed as work and Whites enjoy creating a routine. Don't worry about making training sessions fun.

8. Consider planning sessions at off-peak times; Whites like calm and privacy and will likely appreciate a quieter space. Explain the predictable traffic flow of the facility so they can choose to exercise when crowds are down.

9. Your challenge as a trainer is to address White's need for constant self-improvement, while providing comfort in routines. For example, add intensity to familiar exercises.

10. Advance planning is important to Whites. Advise them as to changes in fitness schedules, disruptions in service, and other routine breakers. If their trusted trainer is leaving, assist in providing a transition to a new trainer.

Keep in Mind:

Whites with Efficiency expect a trainer to have a high level of proficiency and knowledge and will challenge them with tough questions.

Whites with Harmony look for friendly and supportive coaches. They respond best to those who communicate their interest and caring, while at the same time are committed to help them reach their goals.

TOP TEN TIPS FOR COACHING PURPLES

1. Purples apply their own vision and critical thinking to anything they do, so trainers will need to work with them to develop routines according to their vision and goals.

2. Purples enjoy the amenities of a fitness facility and, with advanced planning, will enjoy creating a routine and making use of a well-appointed locker room and spa facilities.

3. Staying in shape is part of what Purples expect of themselves. A trainer can provide value in assisting them to address these expectations

4. Organize a fitness plan into categories, showing that all areas are covered. With their Intuitive nature, Purples see the body/mind/spirit connections. Include this aspect in one of the categories addressed.

5. Purples enjoy routine, but are willing to experiment with new classes and offerings. Who knows—they might incorporate these new offerings into their routine.

6. If not engaging a trainer on a regular basis, Purples enjoy checking in for a "tune up" to be sure they're on track or to take their routine to a higher level.

7. Be aware of Purples' tendency to let their minds drift into internal musings. You may need to provide a constant physical presence, with plenty of eye contact, to keep them focused and attentive to the task at hand.

8. Don't worry about making workouts fun; it's a plus if they enjoy the session, but fitness is about work and improvement.

9. Purples like to control their environment and have strong preferences. If possible, let them choose a location in the gym for their training session.

10. Purples will share feedback about a fitness facility and expect an immediate response.

Keep in Mind:

Purples with Efficiency employ a trainer to help them achieve targeted results with a minimum of wasted effort. The relationship is business-like and impersonal.

Purples with Harmony tend to develop personal relationships with their trainers. They expect a coach to be friendly and enthusiastic about their progress.

REFERENCES AND SUGGESTED READING

Allen, Judy and Susan Brock. *Healthcare Communication Using Personality Type: Patients are Different!* New York: Routledge Press, 2003.

Bayne, Rowan. *Ideas and Evidence: Critical Reflections on the MBTI® Theory and Practice.* Gainesville: CAPT, 2005.

Berens, Linda and Dario Nardi. *The 16 Types, Descriptions for Self Discovery.* Huntington Beach: Telos Publications, 1999.

Campbell, Scott. *A Quick Guide to the Four Temperaments for Peak Performance.* Huntington Beach: Telos Publications, 2003.

Haas, Leona and Mark Hunziker. *Building Blocks of Type.* Huntington Beach: Unite Press, 2006.

Keirsey, David and Marilyn Bates. *Please Understand Me.* Del Mar: Prometheus Nemesis Book Company, 1984.

Kroeger, Otto. *Type Talk at Work.* New York: Dell Publishing, 1992.

Lawrence, Gordon. *People Types and Tiger Stripes.* Gainesville: CAPT, 1993.

Martin, Charles R. *Looking at Type, The Fundamentals.* CAPT, 2001.

Myers, Isabel Briggs. *Gifts Differing.* California: Davis-Black Publishing, 1980.

Myers, Isabel Briggs, Mary H. McCaulley, Naomi L. Quenk and Allen L. Hammer. *MBTI Manual: A Guide to the Development and Use of the Myers-Briggs Type Indicator®*, Third Edition. Palo Alto, 1998.

Myers, Steve. *Influencing People Using Myers Briggs.* England: Team Technology, 1995.

Pearman, Roger R. and Sarah C. Albritton. *I'm Not Crazy I'm Just Not You.* Palo Alto: Davis-Black Publishing, 1997.

Pearman, Roger R. *You: Being More Effective in Your MBTI® Type.* Lominger Publishers, 2005.

Quenk, Naomi L. *Was That Really Me?* Palo Alto: Davis-Black Publishing, 2002.

Roizen, Michael, MD, and Mehmet C. Oz, MD. *You On a Diet: The Owner's Manual for Waist Management.* New York: Free Press, 2006.

Sharp, Daryl. *Personality Types.* Toronto: Inner City Books, 1987.

Spoto, Angelo. *Jung's Typology in Depth.* Rudolf Steiner Publishers, 1995.

Thomson, Lenore. *Personality Type, An Owner's Manual.* Boston: Shambhala Publications, 1998.

Tieger, Paul D. and Barbara Barron-Tieger. *The Art of SpeedReading People, How to Size People Up and Speak Their Language.* New York. Little Brown and Company, 1998.

ABOUT THE AUTHOR

Suzanne Brue, MS, is a researcher, writer, and consultant on the connection between personality and physical exercise. She is a member of The Vermont Governor's Council for Physical Fitness and Sports, and President-Elect of the Association for Psychological Type International (APTi).

Suzanne enjoys a variety of activities including weight lifting, biking, swimming, and yoga. Suzanne is married with three adult children. She and her husband, Nord, divide their time between Burlington, Vermont, and Delray Beach, Florida.

3288272